Speech and Hearing Problems in the Classroom

"This book is particularly concerned with the kinds of speech disorders found among school children and what the classroom teacher can do about them both with and without the assistance of a school speech clinician."

"Parents and teachers may also be involved in a program of reinforcement or reward for the child's use of the language structure being taught. Often programs of parent counseling are a part of the therapy procedure."

"This positive attitude, so vital in the child's life, can be acquired by the child only through his parents' attitude and willingness to help, and through the teacher's ability to acquire and maintain an attitude of friendliness in the classroom."

CLIFFS SPEECH AND HEARING SERIES

PHYLLIS P. PHILLIPS, *Editor*
Head of Speech Pathology
Speech and Hearing Clinic
Auburn University

SPEECH AND HEARING PROBLEMS IN THE CLASSROOM

by

PHYLLIS P. PHILLIPS

Head of Speech Pathology
Speech and Hearing Clinic
Auburn University

CLIFFS NOTES, INC. · LINCOLN, NEBRASKA

Library of Congress Catalog Card No.: 74–78838
ISBN 0–8220–1807–1

Contents

PART 1
AN OVERVIEW

Chapter 1

Introduction

"Speech is civilization itself . . .
it is silence which isolates."

Thomas Mann

Can there by any real doubt that an aspect of human behavior so common, so vital, so often poorly used as speech should be an integral part of the curriculum offered by our schools? With the current emphasis on communication, speech is indeed the very lifeblood of modern existence.

The Responsibility of Schools for Speech Training

Much has been written about the purpose of American education, and the theme that emerges from the writings of most professional educators is that it is to help each child to develop to the maximum of his potential. It then would follow that the schools not only have an opportunity to provide for the special needs of each child but also have a responsibility to do so. The responsibility is not only for the "whole education" of the child, it is also for the education of the "whole child." These concepts of American education are consistent with the basic tenets of democracy that stress the worth and dignity of each individual. Despite a growing conviction that the school must assume a responsibility for the welfare of the child extending considerably beyond simply the development of literacy, some schools still do not make any special provisions for the large number of school-age children with inadequate speech. Speech-handicapped children continue to find it difficult to join the mainstream of activities of the human race because they cannot speak its language.

The tenets of Gestalt psychology and the findings of experimental research all point to the conclusion that the child develops as a whole, and that it is impossible to isolate completely any individual factors involved in his growth and development.

It is being unrealistic to assume that a handicap such as a hearing loss or a speech defect can be ignored on the grounds that it is not of immediate concern to the teacher whose business supposedly is the education of the child. In reality, such a

9

handicap should be of vital concern to the teacher and to the school, because it may well explain why the child is retarded in his studies, is socially immature, or is definitely a behavior problem (1).

Reflecting this basic philosophy, a characteristic of the modern school is the recognition of individual differences and the resultant importance placed on adjusting teaching methods and curricula to meet such differences. Often, however, such individualization is slanted only toward individual abilities, and it must be remembered that children exhibit individual disabilities as well. If a child is to develop to his fullest potential, specific disabilities must be taken into consideration and efforts made to discover and alleviate them.

In this rapidly shrinking world, brought about by improved communication and travel, speech may no longer be taken for granted. Nothing is more basic to education than speech, for without it many normal activities in a highly communicative society are difficult to achieve. School personnel and parents are becoming increasingly aware of the need for all children to develop the ability to communicate their ideas effectively with acceptable speech, voice, and language. This awareness has led to an increased interest in helping children with minor and/or major problems of oral communication. In turn, this growing interest has increased the number of people seeking remediation services. Even so, few normal speakers, other than those in close contact with a speech-handicapped person, realize the impact that a speech handicap has on a person.

Although in Europe the medical profession has taken major responsibility for speech correction, in this country the responsibility has been given to the public schools. There are perhaps three reasons for this. First, the basic philosophy of the American school system certainly indicates that schools provide remediation for the speech-handicapped school population. Second, the school systems are in a position to employ trained speech clinicians. Finally, they have the children during the years when speech correction can be very effective.

Definitions

In any profession there is often terminology that is unique to that profession, and familiarity with that terminology is basic to understanding much of the professional writing. Since the present book is written for professional educators rather than for professional speech pathologists, an effort has been made to avoid overly technical terminology as well as controversial terminology. The author has attempted to choose the simpler, more commonly accepted terms whenever a choice existed. Nevertheless, the definition of certain terms will aid the reader.

The Profession

Since this is a relatively young profession, having grown out of a variety of other disciplines and professions, even those within the profession have had difficulty in agreeing on identification terminology. Although the term *speech pathology* has been accepted as generic for the profession, the term *speech and hearing* has historically been accepted as connoting interest in normal as well as disordered processes of communication, and more recently the terms *communicative disorders* and *disorders of oral communication* have gained wide acceptance (2).

The Professional

Within the profession, there are those who are primarily concerned with research, those whose primary interest is in teaching, and those whose work is primarily concerned with speech remediation—the practitioner. Often coming from varying backgrounds and working in different settings, the professionals also have various identification terminology. The term *speech therapist* is no longer accepted, although in the public schools we find *speech correctionists*, *speech improvement teachers*, *speech clinicians*, and, more recently, *speech specialists* (2). Usually in the clinic or hospital setting, the practitioner is a *speech clinician* or a *speech pathologist*. These terms seem to have more of a medical connotation. In the teaching or research setting we more frequently find the *speech pathologist*, whose title has been applied to the profession.

Defective Speech

Speech has frequently been described as defective when (a) it interferes with communication, (b) it draws unfavorable attention to itself, or (c) it causes its possessor to be maladjusted (3). Perkins says that speech is defective when "it is ungrammatical, unintelligible, culturally or personally unsatisfactory, or abusive of the speech mechanism" (2). Obviously, the term *speech* is not used in a restricted sense. In order to use the term *defective speech* meaningfully, it is necessary to understand the context in which the term *speech* is used.

Speech

Although the term *speaking* is used to identify observable processes of oral language, *speech* is not so restricted. "*Speech* is often used in this technically restricted sense as well as in a broad sense to include covert thinking processes of language and overt phonetic processes of speaking" (2). We may, therefore, use *speech* to refer to the articulated word, or we may use it to refer to the total expression. This may include language, the voice used in speaking, and the rhythm and inflection used. Usually the intent is obvious from the context and little confusion arises in the normal daily use of these terms. The numerous *speech and hearing clinics* throughout this nation serve as evidence of this; they have little difficulty in communicating that they serve individuals with communication disorders other than only defective articulation of words or sounds.

Speech Remediation Services in the Schools

Since 1910, when the Chicago public school system first provided a program of special remedial services for speech-handicapped children (4), both local and state support for such programs have increased substantially. By 1950, thirty state departments of education (5) had established certification requirements for public school clinicians and an estimated four thousand individuals were then employed in such positions (6). In 1974, the number of public school speech clinicians had almost doubled (7).

The addition of speech clinicians to school staffs is an outgrowth of the interest in children's individual needs and of the increased emphasis on improved oral communication. Nevertheless, despite the encouraging advances made in the education of the speech handicapped in the nation as a whole, there are still areas where no specialized speech correction services are available through the school system.

Regardless, however, of the presence or absence of a speech clinician in a school system, the *key* person in the speech development of the school-age child is the classroom teacher. This does not imply that the classroom teacher would provide speech therapy, but rather that he is charged with the responsibility of meeting the speech needs of all children in the classroom. The teacher, cognizant of the significant role that speech plays in a person's ability to become a fully functioning member of this conversant society, must be concerned with speech. Aware, also, of the significant role that he, the classroom teacher, has in the development of clear, pleasing, and efficient speech, the teacher must be prepared to do a great deal of constructive speech teaching himself. This should be in connection with the normal curricular and extracurricular activities in which speech plays a part.

Many young children have the kind of speech and voice characteristics that may be improved through instruction in the classroom; therefore, many schools have begun speech-improvement programs in which the regular teacher has the major responsibility for speech improvement (8). *Speech improvement* refers to the instruction that is provided in the regular classroom for the purpose of improving the oral communication skills of all children; whereas *speech therapy* or *speech correction* refers to the specialized remediation for individual children that takes place outside the curriculum of the regular classroom. The classroom teacher usually has responsibility for speech improvement and the speech clinician provides the speech correction.

Sometimes the speech clinician will engage in some speech improvement with the entire class. In many schools, this is done with the school speech clinician having periodic (perhaps weekly) speech-improvement lessons that may be somewhat in the form of demonstration lessons. The classroom teacher, then, follows up with the remainder of the speech-improvement instruction. Speech-improvement programs, however, are not limited to those schools having the services of a speech clinician, and many classroom teachers initiate and carry out such programs as a part of the daily class schedule.

Realizing the inevitability of teachers' encountering some children with defective speech, it becomes apparent that school personnel must be concerned with how best to meet the needs of the speech handicapped. Phillips (9), in an extensive survey of classroom teachers' attitudes and understandings of speech-handicapped school children, found that the single most significant variable affecting these was if the teacher had had a basic course in speech correction. It therefore appears imperative that teachers become knowledgeable about both the common and the uncommon kinds of speech problems found in the regular school population. The purpose of this book is to provide teachers with understandings that will better enable them to understand and help the speech-handicapped children whom they may encounter. This help will be in the form of recognizing speech problems, making referrals, supporting the work of the speech clinician, and assisting the individual child in appropriate ways. The latter may be any number of concerns, such as helping the child to adjust to his problem, counseling with parents concerning remediation, providing a helpful classroom atmosphere, providing classroom activities aimed directly at aiding the child in correcting his problem, or in providing leadership in securing remediation.

The Classroom Teacher as a Speech Teacher

The classroom teacher is a speech teacher whether he is trained to be or not; indeed, whether he wants to be or not. Both as a speaker and as a listener, he creates an atmosphere either conducive to, or unfavorable to, the development of each child's speech.

Above all from a speech correction point of view, she [the teacher] creates each day a situation in which the child with a speech difficulty tends to be either demoralized or helped not only to improve his speech but also to live gracefully with his problem so long as it persists and to grow as a person through the experience he has with it. . . . The educational leaders, teachers, and speech correctionists of this nation exercise, individually and all together, an influence of fateful importance in the lives of our speech handicapped children . . . (6).

Certainly the large numbers of children enrolled in most elementary school classrooms prohibit the classroom teacher from being able to provide individualized speech correction, even if he should possess the technical skill. Therefore, most of the classroom teacher's efforts must be in the form of speech improvement intended to raise the speech standards of the group as a whole, while giving some assistance to the speech-defective child.

... the classroom teacher enjoys a position of strategic importance with respect to the speech education of her pupils and thereby acquires a responsibility for their speech welfare—a responsibility that cannot be wholly or successfully delegated, even to the special speech teacher (1).

The objective, then, of a speech program in a school is to give *all* children those speech skills that will enable them to meet adequately their EDUCATIONAL, ECONOMIC, and SOCIAL OBLIGATIONS. The function of the classroom teacher is to give continuous training for developing the best speech of which all children are capable. Within the classroom at least four areas are the concern of the teacher: (a) the prevention of speech disorders, (b) general speech improvement for all children, (c) the refinement of speech skills, and (d) the correction of speech defects. Although the teacher will be directly concerned with (a) and (b) above, he will be involved at least indirectly with (c) and (d).

The teacher is important in creating a comfortable atmosphere in the classroom—one into which the speech-defective child can fit without fearing ridicule or rebuke from his classmates (10). It is the intent of the author that this book will serve to help both prospective and practicing teachers to understand better the process of speech—how it develops; what may explain the different rates of development; what may be done to accelerate this development; the various pathologies of speech; and principles of remediation—so that the teacher may be better qualified to cope with the speech needs of all children. This book is particularly concerned with the kinds of speech disorders found among school children and what the classroom teacher can do about them both with and without the assistance of a school speech clinician. The classroom teacher should have some basic understanding of the etiology of the problems as well as of rehabilitative procedures used by the speech clinician. The latter is not intended to equip the classroom teacher with therapy skills, but rather to aid in his understanding of the general principles of therapeutic management so that he may be more supportive of the speech clinician's work and may assist the speech-handicapped child within the limitations of the classroom setting. Furthermore, speech clinicians frequently rely on teacher referral for the identification of children with defective speech. This book should better equip teachers to make such identification. Finally, the concern for effective speech and voice may provide the impetus for some classroom teachers to improve their own oral communication.

Prevalence and Classification

As previously stated, within the school-age population are found children with all degrees of verbal proficiency, from the exceptionally articulate to those whose impairment of oral communication skills is tremendously handicapping. The prevalence at either extreme is small; the majority of children have speech that is adequate. A significant percent, however, have speech that could be described as defective. Among the disorders of oral communication are defective articulation, language, rhythm, voice, and hearing.

Prevalence

Although a number of studies have been conducted in the United States to determine the number of speech-handicapped children, there is considerable variation in the reported results. Studies indicate that from 5 to 25 percent of the school-age population have significant speech disorders. One of the most conservative estimates is that reported by the American Speech and Hearing Association Committee for the 1950 White House Conference, (11), which reports that 5 percent of the population between the ages of five and twenty-one have significant speech disorders. Because of the extensiveness of the survey, this report has continued for a number of years to serve as a point of reference for subsequent studies, most of which tend to place the figure somewhat higher than 5 percent. Based on the majority of recent studies, *it is probably safe to judge that between 8 and 10 percent of the children now enrolled in school exhibit some kind of oral communication disorder.* Although disorders of speech are not respectful of age, sex, or position, the young tend to be especially susceptible (2). Prevalence studies involving adults are less numerous and less reliable than those involving children. Table 1.1 shows the breakdown shown in the Mid-Century White House Conference Report (11).

Such charts should not be taken literally as an accurate prediction of the distribution of speech disorders. There are many opportunities for misinterpretation of such charts and a number of possible explanations for contradictions among reports such as: (a) some surveys are based on reports of classroom teachers or others with little or no training in identifying speech problems, (b) some surveys involve too few children to yield valid conclusions, (c) the basis for judgment varies—a surveyor unfamiliar with a regional dialect may identify dialectal characteristics as articulation problems, and (d) samples vary greatly according to the population being surveyed (12).

Whatever figures are accepted concerning the prevalence of speech disorders, they are impressive enough to cause us to realize that we are

TABLE 1.1

INCIDENCE OF SPEECH DISORDERS ACCORDING TO THE
MID-CENTURY WHITE HOUSE CONFERENCE REPORT (11)

Disorder	Percent of Population
Functional articulation	3.0
Stuttering	0.7
Retarded speech development (language)	0.3
Voice	0.2
Cerebral palsy speech	0.2
Cleft palate speech	0.1
Hearing impairment with speech defect	0.5
TOTAL	5.0

concerned with a significant percent of our population. It has been suggested that, taking the lowest estimate of 5 percent, the number can be visualized in this way. If all of the school-age children in the United States with speech handicaps were brought together in one place they would fill a city the size of Los Angeles. Their number equals or exceeds the populations of twenty-seven states (13).

The frequency of occurrence is, however, not the true measure of the seriousness of the problem. Although their relative numbers are small, cases of stuttering and speech problems associated with cleft palate, cerebral palsy, and hearing disabilities present great difficulties in treatment. Generally, articulation cases respond most easily and quickly to therapy, but there are exceptions to this. Our culture tends to judge articulation and voice defects as being less handicapping than other speech disorders, but in the final analysis the speech-defective individual himself is the only one who can make this evaluation. A tiny lisp may become invested with so much emotional impact that it may dominate an entire lifetime.

Classification

Speech disorders may be classified in several ways, but perhaps the most common grouping is on the basis of symptom; for instance, symptoms observable in articulation, language, rhythm, and voice. This present discussion also includes speech problems associated with cleft palate, cerebral palsy, and a brief discussion of aphasia. Also included are communication problems associated with hearing impairment. Each problem is identified here but dealt with in more detail in Part II of this book.

Articulation Disorders

Articulation is defective when sounds are perceived by the listener as omitted, substituted, or distorted. Sometimes, too, errors are made in which the speaker correctly makes the intended sound but improperly adds another sound. The bulk of all speech disorders are of the articulatory type, making up over three-fourths of the total number. These problems may be so mild that only a professional speech pathologist would notice the oral inaccuracy or they may be so severe that speech is unintelligible. Articulatory defects are variously described by such common terms as:

1. *Baby talk*—speech characterized by the use of sounds often used by the normal child in the early stages of speech development, for example, "tat" for "cat" and "peet" for "feet" or the omission of sounds as "ni" for "knife" or "pate" for "plate."
2. *Lisping*—speech characterized by defective sibilant sounds (*s*, *z*, *sh*, and *zh*, which are often produced as *th*.)
3. *Oral inaccuracy*—a wastebasket term for mild articulatory defects.

These are not the only terms associated with articulatory problems, but they are the ones that the reader will probably most frequently encounter.

Most articulation problems are of the "bad habit" type; thus, with no organic basis, they are usually readily remediable. The seriousness of the problem, however, is not so much in the difficulty of remediation, but rather in the attitudes of many parents and teachers, who may not consider articulation defects to be serious. The assumption is often made that the child will outgrow such speech inaccuracies, and the resultant course of action is NO ACTION. People do not feel this way about articulatory problems with an organic basis, such as those associated with cleft palate or cerebral palsy.

Language Disorders

The language disorder traditionally referred to as *delayed speech* or *delayed language* may be one of the most difficult on which to find agreement both in terms of label and estimated prevalence. The two above terms have been used to describe children whose speech is late in appearing or whose speech development is limited: in other words, deviant language development. This does not mean that these children have normal speech that is just a little late in developing, but rather that there is a disorder in their language development. Oral communication, of course, is only a facet of language, but for the three- or four-year-old, speech is the observable form; hence the emphasis on speech. Perhaps a more accurate term would be *disordered language development*. The reader should keep in mind that whichever of these or other terms he encounters in his reading, he is dealing with a child's "failure to understand or speak the language code of the community at a normal age" (2).

There is considerable discrepancy, too, among studies that report the prevalence of delayed speech and language. While Table 1.1 indicates that only 0.3 percent of the surveyed population exhibited this problem, other writers indicate that as many as 5 percent "have language problems severe enough to interfere with education" (2). The lower estimates may be accounted for somewhat on the basis of visibility. Severe language deficiency may result in the child's non-admission to school; therefore, the child with a severe language disorder may not be among the school surveys. Second, the child who at three may be classified as delayed or deficient in language acquisition but who is beginning to talk before entering school may exhibit speech that sounds immature. This may result in his being classified as having an articulation problem rather than a language problem. It is the residual, then, of the language disorder (immature articulation) that is obvious. Another way of saying this is that there is considerable overlapping between disorders of language development and articulation acquisition.

Stuttering

Speech in which the normal speech flow is disrupted by hesitations, prolongations, and repetitions of sounds, syllables, words, or even phrases is labeled *stuttering*. We all do some hesitating and backtracking, but what the stutterer does is not the normal kind of disruption, such as a speaker's searching for a word. The stutterer knows perfectly well what he is trying to say; yet he finds it impossible to make the smooth articulatory movements necessary for normal speech rhythm. He gets "stuck" on a word or a sound and is unable to go on naturally. Perhaps stuttering can best be described as "abnormal initiation of speech sounds" (2).

Stuttering varies from one individual to another, so that it is impossible to describe observable behaviors except to say that the stutterer exhibits abnormal and uncontrollable repetitions and prolongations that disturb the rhythm of his speech. The other characteristics represent his own individualized modification of the stuttering and may vary from non-existent accessory features to those that are far more disturbing to his speech than his stuttering. These may include eye blinking, head jerking, finger snapping, and the like.

Although the prevalence of stuttering in the general population is not a staggering figure—around 1 percent—it represents one of the most severe speech problems in terms of listener evaluation and in terms of the stutterer's evaluation of the difficulty. The stutterer's speech is disturbing to the listener because the normal rhythm of his speech is disrupted, and the listener feels the stutterer's uneasiness in trying to go on with his message. It is disturbing to the speaker because he is never sure if he can say an intended word without a break in his speech-flow. Stuttering is one of the most baffling problems for researchers, one of the problems most resistant to therapy, and one of the problems least understood by the general public.

Two points that should be made involve the distribution of the stuttering population and problems that may be confused with stuttering. First, since there is considerable evidence that 80 percent of the stutterers recover from or "outgrow" their stuttering, it is obvious that the disorder is far more prevalent among children than among adults (14). Second, a speech-flow disorder that is sometimes confused with stuttering is labeled *cluttering*. This problem has been discussed more in European literature than in this country, but the reader may encounter the term. Although there is considerable disagreement among authorities concerning the nature of the problem, the behaviors can be described. The clutterer sounds as if he were in a hurry. Words seem to tumble over themselves so fast that they become disorganized. The speaker will have repetitions sometimes resembling stuttering, but he generally appears uninhibited about his speech and can improve it when he desires better speech. This is unlike the stutterer, whose speech may worsen when he "tries harder."

Voice Disorders

Voice problems have to do with faults in *pitch*, *quality*, or *intensity*. We expect the pitch of one's voice to be appropriate for his age, size, and sex and are surprised when we hear a large man speaking in a high-pitched voice, or a small woman with a very low-pitched voice. We may not be consciously aware of the quality of a person's voice, yet be able to recognize that person's voice over the telephone. The distinctive quality of each individual's voice allows such identification. Some voices we find pleasing; others may be less so because of a particular quality, such as nasality, harshness, hoarseness, breathiness, or stridency. Intensity refers to loudness, which, of course, should be appropriate to the situation.

Voice problems are perhaps more prevalent than we usually consider. Although Table 1.1 indicates the prevalence of voice problems to be only 0.2 percent of the population, more recent surveys suggest that it is closer to 2 percent. Some of the differences may reflect difficulty in identifying deviant voice characteristics. Since it is sometimes difficult to decide what is normal and what is defective in terms of voice quality, we may tend to ignore a vocal abnormality. Too, voice is so closely associated with personality that we may feel that identifying someone's voice as defective is to do the same for his personality; therefore, we pretend not to notice or we simply accept his voice as a part of his personality. Furthermore, voice problems are frequently not thought of by the layman as forms of speech problems. Classroom teachers, in making referrals to the school speech clinician, usually overlook voice disorders.

Special Problems

Some organic conditions result in speech disorders that may involve any or all of the above-mentioned classifications. Notable among these are cleft palate, cerebral palsy, and aphasia.

Cleft palate is a condition in which the palate or roof of the mouth is not completely closed at birth. The opening may be extensive, reaching from the soft palate through the gum ridge and through the lip; or the cleft may be slight, involving only a portion of the soft palate. A cleft of the lip, too, can be extensive, reaching into the nose or so slight as to be little more than a notch in the lip. Clefts of the lip are usually surgically closed shortly after birth, often with no associated speech problem, unless there is an associated cleft of the palate. Both clefts of the palate and of the lip may be on only one side (unilateral) or on both sides (bilateral).

Clefts of the palate represent a condition relatively difficult to repair so that the child is able to achieve normal speech. Frequently, the child with such a cleft, even after surgery, has difficulty articulating speech sounds that require the buildup of air pressure in the mouth, such as plosives (e.g., *p* sound) and fricatives (for example, *s* sound). The reason for this is not difficult to understand. The child does not have a normal means of closing off the mouth cavity from the nasal cavity. When he tries to build up air pressure in his mouth, the air escapes through his nose. Naturally, this gives his speech the nasal quality that we typically think of as cleft palate speech. In addition to the defective articulation and nasal voice quality, according to many researchers the cleft-palate child may have some language deficit. In addition, the child's unusual efforts to articulate certain sounds may result in some abnormality in his speech rhythm. The speech of the cleft-palate child may vary from normal speech or speech with merely a defective quality to speech that is unintelligible.

Cerebral palsy is a disturbance of the motor function resulting from damage to the brain before, during, or shortly after the birth of the child. The production of normal speech is dependent on normal motor movements for breathing, as well as for articulation. Speech of the cerebral-palsied individual may be normal, but usually it is defective. It tends to be slow, jerky, and labored with faulty rhythm. The fine motor movements necessary for normal articulation may be impossible for the cerebral-palsied child, and he will tend to omit or distort the more difficult consonants. His total speech problem generally encompasses more than articulatory errors, as defective voice quality, faulty rhythm, and some retardation in language acquisition are common.

Aphasia is a language impairment caused by damage to the language area of the brain. Generally, the condition of aphasia is not encountered in the school population. The reader may be familiar with some elderly person whose speech was impaired following a stroke (cerebrovascular accident) or perhaps with a person who has been unable to talk following a head injury, such as one sustained in an automobile wreck. This condition is known as *aphasia*, or *dysphasia* as it may be called. Sometimes the condition is temporary and normal speech returns with time and perhaps speech therapy; sometimes the damage is more-or-less permanent. It should be noted that in these examples the accident to the brain occurred after speech was learned. Brain injury can occur prior to the development of speech. Until recently, such cases were labeled childhood aphasia, but this term is seldom used now. *Specific language disorder, brain injury,* and *minimal cerebral dysfunction* are more common with reference to injury to the preschool-age child.

Hearing Impairment

Speech is learned. Without adequate hearing a child lacks the normal means of learning oral communication. Many hearing problems are so mild that they go undetected; yet they are significant enough to handicap normal articulation. Hearing problems may result in language impairment, faulty articulation, or deviant voice quality. Approximately 3 percent of the school-age children have hearing losses that are educationally significant (interfere with the child's achievement in school). Another 5 percent have impairments that require medical attention, and that may, to some degree, affect speech. About 1 percent of these children require the services of a speech pathologist because of defective speech associated with their hearing impairment (15). Again, figures vary, but whatever figures are accepted, they are impressive enough to warrant thoughtful consideration of the individual problems they represent.

Speech and Success in School

With our awareness of the interrelatedness of the various language skills, it should not surprise us that research indicates some very interesting relationships among speaking, listening, reading, spelling, and also success in school.

Listening

Although listening had received little research attention prior to mid-century, it has been the subject of a tremendous amount of recent investigation. Indications are that children become poorer listeners as they progress through school, that listening ability is related to reading ability, and that listening skills can be taught (16).

The indication that first graders are better listeners than second graders, and that second graders are better listeners than third graders, and on through the grades has raised some questions among school personnel. Do we teach children to become poorer listeners as they go through school? Perhaps in some ways we do. We may bombard the youngsters with so much talk that they have to tune us out for self-preservation. Second, perhaps we teach them early in their school careers that when we have something important to say, we will cue them. We do this inadvertently by prefacing important instructions with carrier phrases such as "Now listen to this" or "Be sure to pay attention to this" or some other cue. Perhaps teachers are not the originators of the cue system; perhaps mothers have taught children this before they come to school—or perhaps it is human nature to need to "be tuned" in. Did not the town crier preface his news with "Hear ye, hear ye," and Longfellow begin his poem with "Listen, my children, and you shall hear"? Nevertheless, such cues serve not only to let the child know when to listen, but also to tell him that the rest of what we have to say is not important, or that it does not merit his effort to listen. And listening *does* require effort. Listening depends on hearing, but the two terms are not synonymous. Listening is the process of interpretation.

Learning to read may be related to listening ability. Bonner (17) found among fifth-grade students a higher correlation between reading ability and listening ability than between reading ability and IQ. Although poor reading does not necessarily indicate poor listening, the child with a reading problem may likewise be a poor listener.

Listening ability can be improved with instruction. This finding has resulted in many colleges adding courses in listening. College-entrance inventories have begun to include a listening test just as a reading or mathematics proficiency test. Those who score low on the former are recommended to take a course in listening just as those with low scores in other skills are recommended for remedial instruction in other areas. Since listening ability is measurable (can be measured by standardized listening tests) and can be modified through instruction, this is an area of consideration for the classroom teacher. It can be a part of the total language program and more specifically of the speech-improvement program.

Reading

For teachers who are constantly striving to meet the needs of the children with reading problems, an awareness that research shows that speech and reading are related, particularly where oral reading is involved, may well stimulate interest in finding a new way to approach the problem of reading difficulties. Moss (18) found that normally speaking children surpass deficient speakers in speed of reading and freedom from errors. This is, perhaps, not difficult to understand. When a child whose speech is very poor is in the traditional reading circle, his unintelligible pronunciations may be corrected by the teacher or by other children, thus giving both the child and his listeners the impression that he is a poor reader. He may make the assumption that he is unintelligent or lacking worth because of his perception of himself in the reading setting with the resultant negative effect on his self-concept and in turn on his performance. It is easy to see that he may, indeed, perform as a poor reader. It is, likewise, reasonable to assume that he may generalize from the oral-reading experience to silent reading; thus, his entire school program may become altered because of an articulation problem.

Obviously, the implications are far more complex than the simplified discussion above. Eames (19) suggested that defects in both speech and reading may stem from the same cause and that therapy for both could be similar and complementary. Jones (20) found that speech-improvement lessons resulted in improved silent-reading achievement scores—this in the absence of any special reading instruction.

Spelling

Ham (21) reported that words that are misarticulated tend to be misspelled even though the spelling error is not related to the type of mispronunciation. In other words, one may expect a child who said "wook" for "look" to spell it the way that he pronounced it. He may indeed misspell the word, but perhaps as "lood" or "lof," suggesting that perhaps articulatory problems may be accompanied by problems in language skills.

Academic Achievement

According to research, children with speech defects tend to be somewhat retarded in their school achievement, having more failures, taking longer to complete the elementary grades, and completing fewer years in school than their more articulate classmates (22). Difficulties noted above in listening, reading, and spelling are possible contributing factors to the speech-handicapped child's lack of success in school, but these cannot be separated from the impact of his self-concept and others' perceptions of him.

Finally, it is not within the scope of this book to investigate all areas of language learning, nor is it the intent of the author to prescribe teaching methods. It is, rather, the intent to point out the significance of speech in the total language-learning process and to indicate the vital role that it plays in the child's academic success. EDUCATIONALLY, SOCIALLY, and ECONOMICALLY, equipping children with efficient speech is a worthwhile goal for the classroom teacher and for the school system as a whole.

Chapter 2

The Nature of Speech

In order to understand what can go wrong with speech development, the reader needs a basic understanding of the nature of speech. This is a subject for an entire book, so only a very cursory description of the basic points will be presented here. Although the term speech may be used in the limited sense that we use the term *speaking* (to identify observable processes of oral language), we often use *speech* in the broader sense including the thinking processes of *language* and the phonetic processes of *speaking* (2). Because of this dual use of the term speech, the terms *speaking* or *talking* will be used in this discussion to indicate the motor act of uttering speech sounds. With these considerations, we could define *language* as the symbolic formulation of ideas according to semantic and grammatical rules and *speech* as a learned system of arbitrary, vocal symbols by which thought is conveyed from one human being to another. This definition of speech implies several things, namely:

1. That it is learned—not instinctive.
2. That it is a system—a code or set of rules.
3. That it is arbitrary—no reason exists for any word (symbol) to mean what it does, or for the system as a whole to have the characteristics that it has.
4. That it is vocal.
5. That it is a function limited to human beings.

True, some animals use signs to call their young, suggest mating, shout danger, and the like, but with a few debatable exceptions, these signs are not speech. Man has some instinctive cries, too, but HIS SPEECH IS LEARNED: instinctive cries are not. A number of writings explore the theories of learning in general and the theories of speech learning in particular. No attempt will be made here to analyze the many theories concerning the development of speech. The reader may consult the Bibliography for suggested readings. Suffice it to say that in spite of the different explanations regarding the origin of speech, one conclusion that is common to all theories is that speech is learned; it does not just happen. Whether the theoretical position suggests that the infant learns speech by imitation or that he has a biological predisposition to learn speech, in one way or another all say that children learn

24

speech. Certainly, this idea is not new. Quintillian, A.D. 90, devoted twelve volumes to *The Education of an Orator*, suggesting instruction from the cradle to the grave (23).

Normal Speech and Language Development

Perhaps no twentieth-century reader would agree with Sir Thomas Browne in his assertion that Adam and Eve spoke Hebrew and that any child reared in solitude would speak that language. Yet the most recent writings concerned with the origin of speech place much emphasis on man's unique ability to speak because of an innate capacity to acquire a language (24). Regardless of the theoretical position taken concerning the basis for language learning, certain developmental landmarks can be traced.

The newborn baby is the most helpless of all animals; yet this new creature already has a past. Past generations, as well as his prenatal care, make him what he is. He is an individual, but he is also an animal except in certain respects—the most notable of which is potential for language acquisition. Basically, the observable progression from non-speech vocalizations to speech may be described in the following way.

Crying Sounds

Speech may be said to be learned through the baby's relations with speaking humans and their reactions to his vocalizations. For this reason, it can perhaps be said that speech and language learning begin with the birth cry (25). This statement in no way suggests that what the baby is vocalizing is some primitive form of speech. The newborn does not cry as a discrete act. Instead, he reacts negatively and violently to his new environment with muscle contractions of his entire body, and the air rushing in and out of his lungs creates the sound of the birth cry. Observe the arms and legs of a crying infant. Consider that similar movements are taking place throughout his body. The sounds occur because his vocal folds are vibrating along with the contractions of other body muscles. This is a reflexive response and in no sense can be interpreted as speech, but usually speaking human beings do respond to him at this time. If the beginning of speech learning can be so pinpointed, then we must conclude that, for better or worse, the process has begun.

The sounds of the newborn are shrill nasalized wails, often indiscriminately made on inhalation and exhalation. He soon learns, however, that he can make more efficient use of his vocal mechanism by taking in a quick gulp of air and controlling the exhalation; thus, he produces louder and longer sounds. This basic control of the vocal mechanism generates the raw material for speech. Too, around the end of the first month the infant begins to make some distinctions in his crying, and his mother soon learns to interpret the distinctions. She can recognize a cry that means "I'm hungry" from one that means "I'm awake" or "I'm wet." This still is not speech, as the infant does not conclude that a specific type of cry will result in a certain response. It is still reflexive vocalization. The young baby spends most of his non-crying time sleeping or eating.

Non-crying Sounds

As the baby begins to sleep less, he likewise learns to be awake without crying. This gives him time to experiment with other forms of vocalizations. Crying, his vocal response to unpleasant stimuli, is inadequate to express all of his responses as he begins to be aware of pleasant stimuli.

Babbling

Somewhere around eight weeks of age, Baby begins to be aware of his non-crying sounds, possibly hearing them but perhaps mainly feeling them. *Babbling*, his vocal response to pleasant stimuli, consists of grunts, gurgles, and sighs, and occurs when Baby is enjoying himself—when he is feeling good. These vocalizations are essentially private, and he usually ceases to coo and gurgle when interrupted by a speaker. His oral activity is mainly associated with eating and swallowing. *All* infants go through this stage—even profoundly deaf ones. Babies the world over vocalize the same sound—the universal repertoire of baby sounds.

Although speech stimulation from birth is considered helpful to speech acquisition, babbling occurs without stimulation. In fact, sometimes oversolicitous parents inhibit babbling by interrupting Baby's every vocal attempt with their own vocal play. The mother should permit the infant to enjoy his private babbling uninterrupted and follow his vocal play with her speech stimulation. Quiet periods such as eating, bathing, and dressing times should also be used for vocal stimulation.

Lallation

Gradually hearing enters, and the sounds of vocal play become more refined. Somewhere around the fourth month, Baby begins to listen to his vocalizations and to repeat the sounds that he makes. This stage is sometimes referred to as *lallation*, and it is at this time that hearing becomes a part of the process. Apparently the infant becomes aware of the sound of his own voice and derives pleasure from its use. Periods, of course, overlap, and some authorities refer to all of Baby's non-crying vocalizations by the one term *babbling*. There are differences, however, in the kinds of vocalizations made; hence the different labels. The observable distinction between babbling and lallation is that while the former consisted of random grunts, gurgles, and sighs, in the next stage Baby tends to find pleasure in recreating sounds that he has just made. He may repeat a syllable over and over for a long time. He seems to listen to himself and to commune with himself in what has been described as a "delightful little fairy language." The distinct pleasure that the baby derives from imitating the sounds that he has made is a fascinating experience for observers, who often interrupt it with their own enthusiasm. Again, parents should provide stimulation by imitating the baby's sounds when he finishes his vocalizing rather than by interrupting his vocal play.

The importance of adequate hearing to this stage of development can be verified because congenitally deaf babies do not progress beyond the babbling stage.

Echolalia

During the second six-month period, sounds become still more refined, and Baby begins to repeat sounds heard in his environment. He experiments with sounds that he recognizes and imitates sounds made by others. This stage is called *echolalia*. Many sound combinations made by the child during this period are misinterpreted as words. It is important for the parents to enter into the vocal play during this stage. The child begins to copy not only the sounds but also the rhythm and inflection of adult speech.

In addition, you will observe that the child is concurrently developing speech comprehension as he gives obvious indications that he understands certain words and phrases, for example, "no, no" or "bye, bye." Many such first understood words are accompanied by specifically repeated gestures. Perhaps the child first learns the gestures, but it is evident that he is developing understanding—receptive language as it may be called. He recognizes both the sound and the meaning but cannot yet verbalize the communication. Likewise, you may note that he understands certain kinds of speech through "tone of voice information." The scolding emphatic tone that accompanies our "no, no" may carry more meaning than the word "no".

During the echolalic stage, the speaker can help the child understand by limiting talking; that is, by using short sentences, much repetition, and accompanying gestures.

Words

Somewhere around the child's first birthday, he probably develops his first true WORDS. Usually these are double-syllable words, such as "mama" and "bye bye" or "bow bow," and usually they consist of easily made sounds such as *m* and *b* in combination with a vowel.

These first true words usually give parents a great deal of pleasure, and in turn parents reward Baby with much stimulation. As previously stated, many accidents are interpreted as words, and with the resultant stimulation, they do become words. For instance, a contented happy baby may be enjoying playing with front-of-the-mouth sounds or even vocalizing while blowing saliva bubbles. An accidentally produced approximation of "mama" will probably result in much attention, stimulation, and socialization from Mother in her efforts to get Baby to "say it again." When Dad comes home, the process is repeated. Baby doesn't understand all of the commotion, but it surely is fun. The tremendous stimulation accompanying that one double syllable enables Baby to recognize it the next time that he accidentally makes it and then to attempt to repeat the sound. When he learns to produce "mama" at will, there is still more reward in the form of attention, stimulation, and socialization. Eventually Baby associates meaning with the word. When he uses it meaningfully, it is a true word.

Most words, however, are learned in the reverse manner. The child learns the meaning of the word before he learns to articulate it. The parent who has stimulated the child with the object "ball" accompanied by the vocal symbol "ball" usually recognizes Baby's production of "bah" as a word. If the parent gives the baby the ball when he makes this gross approximation of the word and the baby appears rewarded (to want the ball), the parent believes that the baby has spoken a word.

Jargon

During the child's second year of life, he continues some of his lallation and echolalia, but also uses the words he is learning. He also engages in a new vocal activity called JARGON, which sounds much like real connected speech, but lacks true words. Anyone who has observed an eighteen-month-old child with a telephone in his hand has probably heard jargon. In this wordless discourse, you may hear questions, commands, amusement, and anger, but it is all communicated through rhythm and inflection. You may hear it, too, as the child "talks" to his Teddy bear or puppy, but in any case, he is practicing for real connected speech.

Perhaps the young speaker thinks that he is doing just what he hears when he listens to adult discourse. If we listen to a foreign newscast given in a language that we studied in school, we may be able to recognize the rhythm and inflection but not be able to understand the message. You may perhaps be able to "pick up" a word or two from the newscast, just as the child may be heard to inject an occasional word into his jargon. This vocal activity usually reaches its peak around eighteen months and usually vanishes by the second birthday.

Speech

The second year of the child's life is the age thought of as the "speech readiness" period and this is the time that we expect a child to begin "to talk." His utterances are a mixture of speech and non-speech vocalizations, but he is generally well on his way to becoming a better communicator. Our observation of his mastery of three components of speech lend credibility to the concept that the infant begins life innately equipped to acquire speech. The child learns (a) to use the sounds of the language to which he is exposed (phonemic competence), (b) the meanings of the words in that language (semantic competence), and (c) the rules of grammar (morphology and syntax).

Although it would be quite a staggering accomplishment, the acquisition of the phonemic and semantic components of speech by imitation could be possible. Learning the grammar of a language by imitation, however, defies such an explanation. The child acquires in approximately a two-year period rules of grammar that his parents would probably be unable to explain or even to state. The mastery of the rules of building words and arranging them into phrases and sentences is a phenomenon observed in young children the world over. How can a child produce a completely original sentence if he learned speech only by imitation?

Consider the toddler whose one-word request, "Cookie" (probably pronounced "tootie") addressed to his mother and understood by her to be "Please, mother, may I have a cookie?" results in his being given a cookie. If, within a few seconds, he again tugs at his mother with the same request, "Cookie," his mother, translating this to "Please, Mother, may I have another cookie?" may respond, "I just gave you a cookie." Here, constructing a sentence completely original with him—one that he has never heard before—the little fellow explains, "Doggie cookie," and his mother likely understands his explanation that the dog ate his cookie.

The two-year-old is a talker. Not all that he says is intelligible even to his mother and still less so to people outside the immediate family. At least one-fourth of his speech, however, should be understood by people outside the immediate family. He makes many mistakes in his articulation, but the most important learning that is taking place during the period from two to four years is the development of rhythm. He has learned many words, yet they often do not come easily for him. His connected speech is characterized by repetitions, stops, and prolongations that disturb expected rhythm patterns, but, given time, he learns through practice how to string words together as his more fluent elders do.

The two- to four-year-old develops fluency and learns to articulate more sounds. He becomes more precise in putting sounds into words and continues to increase his vocabulary. Parents come to think of him as a talker; they tend to expect more fluency than he is sometimes capable of achieving; and they tend to cease to be the exceptional teachers they were when he was first learning a few words. At any rate, the rapid progress in acquiring articulatory skills diminishes around four years and appears to be somewhat at a stand-still for many children until they enter school.

By eight years of age, articulation skills are mature. This means that articulation should be 100 percent errorless. See Chapter 3 for a description of the age and order in which sounds are learned by children.

Inner, Receptive, and Expressive Language

The sequence in which language is learned has been described as beginning with the development of inner language, followed by receptive language, and finally by expressive language (26).

Inner Language

Inner language involves the understanding of the meaningfulness of objects, their use, and their relationships. A deaf child with normal intelligence who has been taught no form of receptive or expressive language would demonstrate his inner language in the appropriate use of objects. For instance, although he would not know the symbol "chair," he would understand "chairness" (If I may use such a term). He would know that he can sit in the chair, climb on it, move it, and use it to make him tall enough to reach a high object. Inner language is often tested clinically in non-speaking children by presenting a doll house with furniture and figures. Observations are made of the meaningful way in which the child plays with the objects and figures. If inner language is prerequisite to further language development, then we could not expect a child who had not developed some inner language to be taught expressive language.

Receptive Language

Receptive language is the ability to decode messages—or to understand language. When a mother makes a request of a baby who has not started talking, such as "Give Mommie a kiss" or "Give Mommie the ball," and the little one responds appropriately, we are observing his receptive language ability. Probably the first evidence of this is accompanied by gesture. When the mother holds out her hands and says, "Want to go bye, bye?" or "Want to get down?" or "Want to come to Mommie?" Baby may respond to the gesture. Eventually, however, he attaches meaning to the words. When we talk about receptive language, we are usually thinking of understanding words—spoken, written, and sign language. Understanding what one hears and understanding what one reads are both examples of the use of receptive language. The same is true for the deaf who understand sign language. Our receptive vocabularies are always larger than our expressive vocabularies.

Expressive Language

Expressive language is the ability to express ideas or messages to others. When the young child looks toward the refrigerator and says "wawa " he is using expressive language. He is saying, "I want some water" just as communicatively as his grandmother who may say, "I'll have a cup of tea, please"—each expression appropriate for the language-learning level of the speaker.

Other forms of expressive language are the sign language of the deaf, codes, and writing. If such a hierarchy of language learning can be visualized, then it would seem reasonable not to expect a child with a reading problem (receptive language) to do well in creative writing (expressive language).

Summary

The child's speech and language development, although altered by many factors within himself and his environment, basically follows a pattern of development. You cannot use a clock or calendar to determine exactly when a particular child will reach a certain stage, but you can generalize about his progress. Table 2.1 gives a basic outline of these landmarks.

TABLE 2.1

CHRONOLOGY OF CHILD'S SPEECH AND LANGUAGE DEVELOPMENT

Age	Activity
Newborn	Birth cry
Birth to one month	Undifferentiated crying
One to two months	Differentiated crying
Two months to five months	Babbling
Five months to eight months	Lallation
Eight months to twelve months	Echolalia
Twelve months	First true words
Twelve months to twenty-four months	Jargon
Two years to four years	Practicing fluency
Six years	Completely intelligible speech
Eight years	Mature articulation

The Communicative Process

The above explanation of how the normal infant learns to talk considers only what we hear and the chronology of the events. Communication is a complicated process that should be understood by anyone concerned with the correction of faulty speech or language. Physiologically, the communicative process can be described in six steps: innervation, respiration, phonation, resonation, articulation, and audition or hearing. A cursory look at each function should help provide a basis for understanding the entire process.

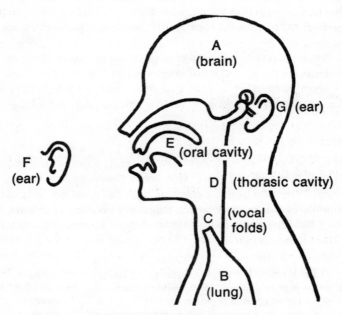

Figure 2.1. The Communicative Process

(A) speech impulse originates in the brain; (B) lungs provide the air supply; (C) voice is formed at the vocal folds; (D) the sound is resonated through the throat and head cavities; (E) articulation is achieved in the oral cavity; (F) the ear of the listener receives the sound; (G) the ear of the speaker provides auditory feedback to the speaker's brain.

Innervation

The speech act is directed and coordinated by the central nervous system. This system includes the brain, in which the speech model is stored and from which the message is encoded, as well as the nerve pathways along which the message travels.

Respiration

The controlled air flow essential for phonation is achieved through the respiratory process of inhalation and exhalation. The rhythm of inhalation-exhalation for life function (a 1:1 ratio) is altered for speech purposes so that the speaker takes air into his lungs in a quick gulp and slowly controls the exhalation phase for phonation. He synchronizes his breathing to make speech more efficient and to enhance the meaning of his utterances. Breath is the sum and substance of the sounds we make in the throat.

Phonation

After the breath is expelled from the lungs via the bronchial tubes, it passes through the trachea (windpipe), at the top of which rests the larynx (voice box). See Figure 2.2. The larynx consists of a group of cartilages, the largest of which can be located by the following simple procedure. Place your finger just below your chin and move it down your neck until it hits a small depression or notch. This is the top of the front cartilage (thyroid cartilage) of the larynx. The vocal folds are attached just behind and below this notch.

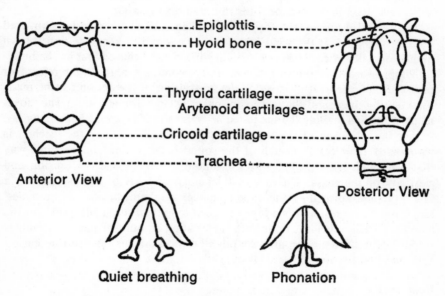

Figure 2.2. The Larynx (above) and vocal folds (below)

From here, extending back along each side wall of the thyroid cartilage, they slope slightly downward and are attached posteriorly to two small ladle-shaped and movable cartilages (arytenoid cartilages). These two small cartilages sit atop a signet-ring-shaped cartilage (cricoid cartilage), which is actually the top ring of the trachea. If you hold your finger where you have located the notch and swallow, you will feel the larynx move up as you utilize your protective mechanism for keeping the swallowed matter from entering your windpipe. Since the larynx of an adult male is considerably larger and usually more prominent than that of a female, you can make use of this prominence in helping locate the larynx. Observe a particularly prominent Adam's Apple of someone as he swallows. You will see it bob up and down as the normal swallow function operates.

In quiet breathing, the vocal folds are apart in an inverted V-shape, together at their anterior attachment (at the notch of the thyroid cartilage) and apart at their posterior attachment (to the artenoid cartilages). See Figure 2.2. For phonation the speaker brings the folds together while allowing exhaled air to build up some pressure beneath them. The folds are held together, but not tightly enough to prevent their being blown apart by the force of the exhaled breath stream. This blowing apart of the folds releases some of the pressure, and they regain their closed state, again building up pressure. The above description is an extemely simplified explanation of the action involved in setting the folds into audible vibration.

The action of the vocal folds has been likened to a swinging door buffered by a strong wind. If the wind is not strong enough to keep the door blown open, you will notice a constant opening and closing caused first by the build-up of pressure that blows it open, and second, by a resultant release of pressure that allows it to close. A demonstration of the action can be made by imitating the sound that a person makes when extremely cold. The movement of the lips making the suggested *brrrrrrrr* sound is somewhat analogous.

It is the vibration of the vocal folds that, when heard by the listener, is recognized as voice. The pitch of the sound is determined in the same way that any pitch is controlled—by the amount of mass and the tension and elasticity of the mass. The larger, thicker vocal folds of adults produce a lower pitched voice than the child's smaller mechanism, just as the males' larger mechanism produces a lower pitched tone than the smaller folds of the female. Likewise, what is done with the existing amount of mass determines pitch. Tighten the tension and the pitch becomes higher; loosen the tension and the pitch becomes lower.

Resonance

Without resonators, the sound generated by the vibrating vocal folds would be inefficient, just as the sounds from bowed violin strings would be rather pitiful without the resonance box beneath. Resonance is the building up or damping of sounds. Resonators do not create sound; they take sound that has already been produced and modify it. Without resonance, the sound made by vocal-fold vibrations would be something like that of a carnival noisemaker.

There are three primary resonators in the speech mechanism: the mouth (oral cavity), nose (nasal cavity), and throat (pharyngeal cavity). The most variable of these is the oral cavity. The English language is essentially an oral language, since most of the sounds are resonated in the oral cavity. Vowels, the carriers of sound, are formed by altering the size and shape of the resonating cavity. A sentence written solely with vowels can easily be read aloud and heard; yet, there would be no meaning to the sounds, for example, ---ee -i--- --ou--- --ei- -u---e-. As you can see, there is the possibility of ample sound, but no meaning. Although we have only five vowel letters in our alphabet, we use more than five vowels in our speech. The Table 2.2. gives our commonly used vowels written in the orthographic symbols employed by dictionaries followed by a key word to help you identify each vowel sound.

TABLE 2.2

THE VOWEL SOUNDS

Symbol	Key Word	Symbol	Key Word
		Vowels	
1. ē	meat	8. ō	sew
2. ĭ	sit	9. o͝o	full
3. ā	cake	10. o͞o	moon
4. ĕ	let	11. ûr	word
5. ă	cat	12. ĕr	mother
6. ä or ŏ	father	13. ŭ	hut
7. ô	saw	14. ə (schwa)	ago (any unaccented vowel)
		Diphthongs	
1. ī	sigh	3. ou	cow
2. oi	boy	4. ū	use

If you pronounce this list of vowels beginning with the first sound, *ē*, you will notice a progressive alteration of the oral cavity beginning with your tongue forward and high. As you move through the vowels, your mandible (jaw) is dropped lower and your tongue lowers and moves back until the most open sound, *ä*, is formed. From this position, your mandible closes gradually and your lips become more rounded as your tongue moves back and up until the highest back vowel, *o͞o*, if formed. The vowels having an "*uh*" or "*er*" sound are formed in the middle of your mouth. Diphthongs are formed by making a sound as you move from one mouth position to another, as in the *ī* sound. You assume the position to form an *ä* and move to the position to form an *ē*. The *ī* sound is made as you change positions. Figure 2.3 gives these vowels in a schematic drawing of the mouth placement for each vowel sound.

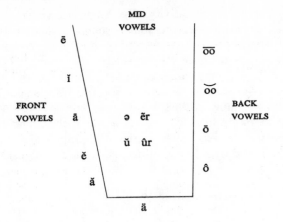

Figure 2.3. Position of vowels

Articulation

Articulation is the process of forming meaningful oral symbols by the manipulation of the articulators—the tongue, lips, lower jaw, teeth, and soft palate. The airstream or sound is modified in such a way that certain characteristic sounds called consonants are made. Some are voiced and some are unvoiced. They constitute a collection of grunts, hisses, pops, and the like, and serve as links for the vowels. Unlike the vowels, which are easily vocalized audibly, consonants may be difficult to say aloud in isolation. Also unlike vowels, the meaning of a sentence can be interpreted simply by seeing the consonants, for example, Thr-- g-rls br--ght th--r l-nch-s. The meaning is apparent, but read that string of consonants aloud! Articulation, then, gives meaning to our phonation. There are twenty-five consonant sounds in our language. Many of them are cognates (pairs) which means that two consonants may be produced in exactly the same manner with one exception—one will be voiced and the other unvoiced, as *b* (voiced) and *p* (unvoiced) or *z* (voiced) and *s* (unvoiced). English consonant sounds are presented in Table 2.3 in the same manner as the vowel sounds with the orthographic symbol and a key word for identification. Note that sounds such as *th* and *sh* are single consonants, not blends. Note also that there are no sounds for three of our consonant letters, the *c*, *q*, and *x*.

Audition

Audition, or hearing, is the final step in the communicative process. If the reason for speech is to communicate thoughts, then there must be a receiver

TABLE 2.3

THE CONSONANT SOUNDS

Symbol	Key Word	Symbol	Key Word
1. p	pencil	13. sh	ship
2. b	box	14. zh	treasure
3. t	top	15. ch	chalk
4. d	dog	16. j	jam
5. f	fan	17. h	hat
6. v	vase	18. y	yellow
7. k	cat	19. m	money
8. g	gate	20. n	nose
9. th (voiceless)	bath	21. ng	ring
10. th (voiced)	this	22. w	water
11. s	sing	23. hw	what
12. z	buzz	24. l	lamb
		25. r	run

of the spoken message; therefore, hearing must take place. As the articulated sound leaves the speaker it travels through a medium, usually air, and impinges on the eardrum of the listener, setting up a series of events that results in the listener's hearing the message. Figure 2.4 shows a schematic drawing of the hearing process.

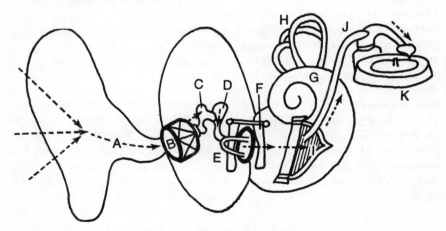

Figure 2.4. The hearing process

Essentially what happens is as follows. The sound waves enter the ear canal (A) and hit the eardrum (B). This membrane is extremely sensitive and can be set into vibration with a minute amount of sound pressure. The vibrating eardrum causes the attachments within the middle ear to be set into motion also. The attachments are three small bones called the ossicles, with the common names of hammer (C), anvil (D), and stirrup (E). The stirrup is set with the footplate in the membraneous part of the inner ear called the oval window (F). The complicated snail-shaped cochlea portion (G) of the inner ear has to do with hearing, while the semicircular canals portion (H) has to do with the sense of balance. The inner ear is filled with a fluid in and around the labyrinthine structures within the cochlea. The movement of the footplate of the stirrup creates movement of the fluid, which in turn sets up movement of the vibrating membrane (I) in the cochlea and results in activation of nerve endings. These nerve endings send the message of sound waves along the auditory nerve (J) to the brain (K), where the sound is interpreted or heard by the listener.

THE COMMUNICATIVE PROCESS—what a complicated sequence of events. Small wonder that there are infinite chances for error!

Speech as an Overlaid Function

Speech is often described as an overlaid function. This means that the body has no speech apparatus per se, but that organs having specific biological functions have been used to produce speech; that is, their biological or life function has been overlaid with the speech function. The purpose of this discussion is not to decide if man was created with organs intended for speech or if he has usurped the use of other organs for this purpose. The description is presented simply to focus on the very complicated nature of speech and the many ways in which normal function can be disrupted. The overlaid function theory can be explained quite simply, as follows.

1. An airstream expelled in a controlled fashion from the lungs is essential for speech. Air in the lungs performs the life function of supplying oxygen to the bloodstream. Seldom is there conflict between the two functions. If conflict occurs, however, the life function always takes precedence over the speech function. We have all viewed some event such as when a swimmer who has just broken a world record is hauled from the pool panting for breath as a sports announcer shoves a microphone before him and asks him how it feels to have set such an incomparable record. The happy swimmer, with his opportunity for a television debut, can do nothing more than pant loudly into the microphone. His body's need to replenish its oxygen supply leaves little opportunity for speech.

2. A second requisite for speech is the vibration of the vocal folds located within the larynx, which sits atop the trachea. The primary function of the

larynx is to prevent foreign matter from entering the trachea. Anyone who has tried to eat a cracker and talk at the same time knows what happens when we defy nature's intent and try to use the mechanism for two functions simultaneously. The life function takes precedence. The story must wait until the crumb has been expelled.

3. Necessary, too, for speech are the cavities that resonate the sound created by the vocal-fold vibration. The principal resonators are the mouth, nose, and throat. The latter two are primarily passages through which air enters and leaves the body. The mouth is used primarily for the intake and mastication of food. Obviously, we cannot use these resonators to amplify and modify our voices when we are chewing, drinking, or inhaling.

4. Finally, the articulators serve dual functions. We use the tongue, palate, lips, and teeth to modify the sounds and form them into meaningful symbols. Their primary function, however, is the ingestion, mastication, and swallowing of food and drink.

It can be hypothesized, then, that the speech function has been added, or is overlaid—that the biological functions are primary. Lyle V. Mayer (27) says that such a theory is as fanciful as it is fascinating—that speech was not given man as an afterthought but that man was provided with a mechanism designed for a double purpose. Regardless of the theoretical position you accept, it is not absolutely precise to say that speech is an overlaid function. Biologically, it may appear so, but man's speech apparatus and his need for speech have doubtless emerged together. Man's need for a form of communication by which he could exert a measure of control over his environment provided the impetus for the development of language; his use of language provided the means of developing and refining a complicated mechanism for its production. Certainly, the mechanism of twentieth-century man is more speech-adapted than that of early caveman, just as other parts of our bodies have adapted to centuries of specialization.

Speech as a Servosystem

A speech model may aid in understanding the process involved in correcting a speech error. Many attempts have been made to fractionate speech and show how the many parts are interwoven. Such models may be helpful in explaining (a) how speech is learned, (b) how the production of speech sounds is controlled, (c) why there are vocal errors and vocal inefficiencies, and (d) how new vocal patterns may be substituted for old ones.

A model of speech as a servosystem (28) may aid our understanding of the complicated process of monitoring what we say. By definition, a servosystem (a thermostat is an example) must (a) provide feedback of output to the place of control, (b) provide comparison of output and input, (c) provide manipulation of the output-producing device so as to cause the output to have the same functional form as the input, and (d) be a closed-loop system—that is, it has no beginning and ending but is continuous. Figure 2.5 presents a schematic drawing of the speaker and listener.

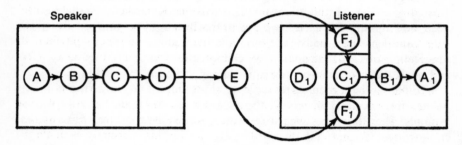

Figure 2.5. Model of Speaker and Listener

The signal originates in the storage area of the brain (A) and is encoded into an intended message also in the brain (B). It is then carried via the neurological system (C) to the speech mechanism (D), where acoustic events are created in the conducting medium, usually air (E). From here it bypasses the speaker's speech mechanism (D_1) and enters his ear (F_1), where it is carried via his neurological system (C_1) to his brain, where the message is decoded (B_1) and finally perceived (A_1). Figure 2.6 shows the same process without the listener. In this model you see the closed-loop servosystem of the speech mechanism.

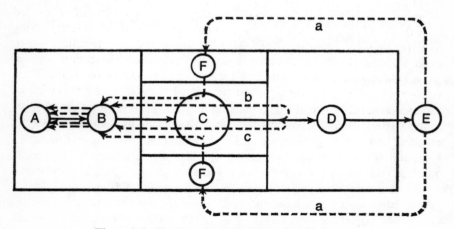

Figure 2.6. The Speech Mechanism as a Servosystem

The speaker, too, hears his own message as it enters his ears (F) and is carried back through his neurological system (C) to the brain (B), where the decoded message is compared (A) with the intended outgoing message. This is auditory feedback (a). If error has occurred, correction can take place. Therefore, we see that we have in the storage area of our brains the "pattern" for the words we may use, and we are able to monitor and correct our productions by this comparison provision. Kinesthetic (muscle sense) feedback (b) and tactile (sense of touch) feedback (c) also go from the speech mechanism via the neurological system to the brain, where they contribute to the comparison and correction. We expect our speech production to "feel right" as well as to "sound right."

The ear now emerges as one of the more important components in the speech mechanism. It has two functions—ESTIMATION and CONTROL. We use our hearing to estimate what others say; we use it to control what we say. If you ask a person to say the word "pay," he uses his hearing to estimate the word according to what he heard or understood you to say; when he repeats the word he uses his hearing to control what he says. A correlate of this would be a set of scales at the market. If you want to buy some apples that sell for $x¢$ per pound and ask for 5 pounds, the merchant uses the scales to control the amount of apples that he sells you. If, on the other hand, you pick up a bag of apples selling for the same price per pound and ask how much the entire bag costs, the merchant then uses the scales to determine how much you owe.

In brief and greatly simplified, the servosystem theory of speech postulates a center in the brain in which comparison can be made of the intended outgoing message (thought) with the actual physiological and acoustical characteristics of the message, relayed by the body's sense organs as it is being produced. When attempting to modify a person's habitual or learned articulation of a certain word, one must consider the feedback. Merely telling him that "candy" does not begin with a t sound and then teaching him to make the desired k sound does not usually consistitute correction. One of the major difficulties encountered is that he has a model of the word in the storage area of his brain for the word articulated "tandy," and that is what he *encodes*; in turn, he decodes "tandy" as "correct," or matching the encoded model. The correction of speech errors will be discussed in the following chapter.

PART II
DISORDERS OF ORAL COMMUNICATION

Chapter 3

Articulation Disorders

Of all the speech problems encountered by the classroom teacher, none will be found with greater frequency than those of the articulatory type. Articulation disorders make up over three-fourths of all speech problems, and over half of this number are misarticulations of the s sound. When the articulation problems associated with cleft palate and cerebral palsy are added to the above figure, we can safely assume that approximately 90 percent of all speech problems are articulatory in nature.

Although the incidence figure is impressive, we find parents, teachers, and speech clinicians who view defective articulation as a mild or simple problem. Perhaps the very frequency of its occurrence causes us to accept misarticulations more than we do a less frequently occurring disorder such as stuttering. Because of the many articulation problems that the classroom teacher encounters and because of our sometimes complacent attitude toward such errors, we should carefully determine what constitutes an articulation error.

Errors of Articulation

Articulation is defective when speech sounds are not produced in an accepted manner. Errors commonly occur in the form of omissions, substitutions, and distortions. Sometimes the addition of a sound such as an "uh" after a word constitutes an articulation error. The severity of the defect is measured in terms of the intelligibility of the speaker's speech. If you have tried to understand a very young child whose speech was filled with omissions and substitutions, you realize how difficult it can be to get the message. With the small child we would think little about such errors of articulation; but with an adult we would view them as a severe problem. All too often the erroneous assumption is that the adult with an articulation problem is uneducated or mentally retarded. Why else would he mispronounce so many words? The total impact of even a mild problem may be very significant.

Omissions

If a speaker omits sounds that are present in normal pronunciation, he has an articulation problem characterized by omissions. Of all types of articulatory errors, omissions are the most severe, since they impair intelligibility to the greatest degree. It is extremely difficult to understand a person who omits many sounds—the more sounds omitted, the less intelligible his speech.

Omitting sounds in words is characteristic of young children just learning to talk. They especially omit final sounds, and very small children may use no final consonants. Omissions are also characteristics of the speech of many poorly educated people and/or the mentally retarded. As children grow older and learn to articulate more accurately, they may learn to include the endings of words; yet, they may have difficulty in putting consonant sounds together in blends such as the *st* in "stove" or of the *pl* in "play." The child who first says "tow" for "stove" may proceed to "tove" for "stove." Usually, children are inconsistent in their omissions, since they are in the process of learning; therefore, inconsistency indicates a better prognosis for correction than does consistency. In other words, consistency of misarticulations indicates that the speaker has not learned a specific pronunciation; thus, such problems are usually more difficult to correct than are the ones made inconsistently.

Substitutions

Sometimes a speaker appears to substitute one sound for another—to substitute incorrect sounds for ones that are normally heard. In the case of the small child, he probably uses a learned sound for one that he has not learned, or more specifically, one that is similar or "heard alike" to him. In listening to his speech you will hear many "front-of-the-mouth" sounds such as *t* used for "back-of-the-mouth" sounds such as *k*. A child whose speech is described as "baby talk" may use primarily front-of-the-mouth sounds in his speech. Here again, this speech behavior is characteristic of young children, and they are generally inconsistent in their substitutions. Older children and adults tend to be more consistent and more resistant to change. Not all substitutions follow the pattern described. Sometimes a person has not learned how to make a certain sound; sometimes the substitution is learned, since speech models in the speaker's environment use that substitution; sometimes a child learns a few sounds and uses them for all others.

Although the term "substitution" has been used, it is doubtful if this is actually what the child is doing. More specifically, he is being much more tolerant of a wider range of variability in sound production; that is, he accepts one sound for several. Perhaps, in many cases it would be more nearly correct to say that he has not yet learned to make fine discriminations between sounds that have similar characteristics. For instance, the child who uses a *t* for the *k* sound may not actually be substituting a *t* for the *k*, but rather be interpreting the *k* as a *t* because of the similarities of the two sounds. Each of these sounds is a voiceless consonant made by stopping the breath stream with the tongue and then quickly releasing it, making a little puff of air. The difference is in the placement of the tongue. If you will make these two sounds yourself, you will see the similarities. For the *t*, the front of your tongue is pressed against your alvealor (gum) ridge and then quickly released, but for the *k* you use the back of your tongue against your velum (soft palate) to block and then release the air. Therefore, it may be said that using *t* for *k* is not an error of substitution, but rather of not quite getting all of the *distinctive features* of certain sounds.

It is not within the scope of this book to investigate the theoretical basis for the use of inappropriate phonemes (sounds), but certain observations concerning remediation are pertinent. Errors such as the one just described are not considered as severe as errors involving the substitution of a sound for one that has more than one different distinctive feature, for example, *m* for *t*. In other words, not all substitutions are equally abnormal.

Speech is difficult to understand when it contains both omissions and substitutions or when it contains numerous substitutions, especially unexpected ones. For instance, "tandy" is readily understood to mean "candy"; whereas, "matty" would not be judged to mean "candy" unless context or gesture provided meaningful clues. Substitutions are often associated with non-standard speech or with low intelligence.

Distortions

Distortions occur when the correct sound is approximated but not closely enough to be normally accepted. Although we allow some variability in the placement of articulators from one production of a specific sound to another production of it, we do not tolerate much alteration. If articulators are placed almost correctly, but not quite, and the resultant sound is slightly different from the accepted model, then the sound is distorted. We notice distortions more in older children and adults than in young children. Usually, speakers are fairly consistent in their distortion of a sound.

Distortions are less noticeable than substitutions and usually do not impair intelligibility. The speaker can be understood, but unfavorable attention is drawn to the way that he speaks. The sound most commonly distorted is the *s*. For instance, an *s* may be produced in a manner that makes it sound "slushy" or "wet," in a manner that makes it resemble a "th," or so forcefully that it is a whistle. The produced sound, therefore, is perceived by the listener as being not quite an acceptable *s*. The *z*, *sh*, *ch*, *v*, and r are also frequently distorted. We are not talking about such pronunciations as "jist" and "git." These are non-standard pronunciations involving incorrect vowels and are usually associated with dialectal speech patterns.

Causes

The child with an articulation disorder is unable to produce consistently and effortlessly the ordinary, accepted sound patterns of speech (12). Therefore, his speech sounds differ from those of the normally speaking child. Why does a child learn to talk in this way? Why does one such child go through the normal misarticulations of a beginning talker and mature to errorless articulation at an early age, while another child with similar environment and speech stimulation develops speech characterized by numerous articulation errors and never achieves errorless articulation without professional assistance? The answer is not simple.

Much is not known about a child's speech-sound discrimination development, but there seems to be some merit to the thesis that "articulation errors represent, for the most part, the incorrect learning of the phoneme system of the language" (29). Causes of articulatory disorders are not easy to explain. They are complex and often obscure. In general, known causes may be divided into certain broad classes such as: (a) constitutional, (b) faulty learning, and (c) emotional maladjustment.

Constitutional Factors

Some of the more severe organic conditions will be discussed separately under headings of cleft palate, cerebral palsy, and hearing disorders. The following may also have an adverse effect on articulation proficiency.

Dental Abnormalities

Good teeth are important to good chewing, to a winsome smile, and also to normal articulation of certain sounds (13). Although important to clear articulation, good dentition does not insure good speech, nor does poor dental alignment necessarily indicate that a person will have articulatory errors. Many people learn to compensate for dental irregularities with amazing results. Consider the children who lose their two front teeth. Some immediately develop articulatory errors, but most do not (30). Dental irregularities may well contribute to articulatory defects, but other factors such as intelligence, creativity, and adequate auditory feedback must also be considered.

Tongue Abnormalities

Since the tongue is the most important articulator, it is important to speech. The term "tongue tied" is frequently heard with reference to articulation errors. Laymen frequently use this term to describe all defective speech and appear to feel that in all articulation cases a physical handicap exists that prohibits the speaker from correctly producing certain sounds. As a result, many purely functional (non-organic or bad habit type) articulation errors are accepted with no effort toward remediation.

There is a condition called "tongue tie" in which the frenum of the tongue, the web of skin underneath the front part of the tongue, is abnormally short. Obviously, if it is too short, it literally holds the tongue down on the floor of the mouth. This results in misarticulations, since the tongue is not free to perform some of the gymnastics necessary for proper articulation. However, if a child could nurse and if he can stick out his tongue, he is not tongue tied.

Frequently, someone attributes poor speech to an excessively large tongue. This is possible, but rare. More often than not such an observation is made of a person who sits with his mouth open allowing his tongue, which is a mass of muscle usually filling the oral cavity, to protrude. Frequently, a child in a class for the mentally retarded is described as having poor speech because of an abnormally large tongue. The child's poor muscle tonus and low mentality contribute to his assuming the open-mouth posture with the resultant protruding flabby tongue. The same open-mouth posture may be assumed by a child with enlarged adenoids because his normal air passageway for breathing is not open.

It is easy to understand why an observer may associate poor articulation with a tongue that appears too large for a child's mouth. Certainly a person with extremely poor muscular coordination may have difficulty in articulating sounds because of his inability to make the rapid fine motor movements necessary for normal speech. A person with a slight paralysis may be a good example. The dysarthric speech of the person who has a motor speech problem resulting from damage to the motor area of the brain is another.

In spite of the importance of the tongue to articulation, there is evidence that people can articulate adequately even without a tongue. The author has an audio tape recording of a speaker who had his tongue removed surgically so that there was not a vestige of tongue tissue left; yet his speech is perfectly intelligible. The point is that tongue abnormalities certainly may contribute to misarticulations but do not necessarily cause them.

Tongue Thrust

A neuromuscular syndrome receiving considerable attention in the last decade or so is known as tongue thrust, or reverse swallowing. This is a condition in which the child thrusts his tongue forward during swallowing. He may also thrust his tongue against the front teeth during rest. Pressure from the constant pushing of the tongue against the front teeth and dental arch may cause dental irregularities. The resultant open bite allows the tongue to protrude between the teeth and frequently results in a distortion of the sibilant sounds. Orthodontists are concerned with the problem of tongue thrusting because of the dental problem created; speech pathologists are concerned because of the frequently associated articulation problem (lisping).

Other Oral Irregularities

Any malformation of oral structures may contribute to articulatory errors. Sometimes, an unusually high, narrow hard palate makes it difficult for the speaker to effect the contact between his tongue and hard palate necessary for some sounds. A palate can be so vaulted that the bony structures invade the nasal cavity, creating an obstruction and causing the speaker's voice to be denasal. Although we often associate denasality with a voice problem, it may be considered an articulation problem, since the speaker cannot articulate the three nasal sounds: *m, n,* and *ng.*

Usually lips are adequate for speech, although sometimes children do not appear to use their lips with much agility. This is usually the lazy-mouth type of speech, and attention given to open-mouth exercises and clear speech may help the child to realize the need to use his lips adequately in speech production. Mouth injuries also may contribute to articulation errors.

This is not an exhaustive listing of constitutional causes, but it includes the most commonly discussed ones. The primary consideration here is that, although structural abnormalities may contribute to articulation errors, it is difficult to say that they are the cause. For every case cited as being caused by a structural abnormality, someone can cite a case with an equal or worse structural problem who has perfect articulation. Avoid looking too hard for constitutional causes.

Faulty Learning

For the majority of articulation problems, no organic basis can be found. There may, of course, be organic factors such as the ones mentioned above that could be considered as contributing factors rather than direct causes. Most articulation problems are the result of faulty learning; they are of the bad habit type. Such speakers need special retraining to acquire normal speech. Two of the more significant causal factors are (a) poor speech models and (b) lack of stimulation and motivation. Articulation is learned from models. Naturally, if a child learns fom a poor model, his speech will reflect this. The lack of stimulation and motivation may result in poor speech for a number of reasons. Often, infantile speech persists because there is no motivation to change. If the baby talk is accepted and never corrected, there is little reason for the child to realize that his speech is non-standard. All too frequently, not only is there no motivation to change, but there is positive reinforcement to retain the baby talk. Parents, thinking that it sounds cute or wanting their child to stay a baby, reward the baby talk and use it when talking to the child. Sometimes such causes may be apparent; often they are not determined.

The author was concerned about the poor therapy progress of a college student with a severe articulation problem. In the absence of any apparent constitutional basis for the problem, one had to wonder why such a bright young man would have developed such poor articulation and why he would persist in using almost unintelligible speech. His college roommate helped supply the answer after spending a weekend in the young man's home. The roommate was astonished at the family's speech and reported, "His entire family sounds just alike. I couldn't understand any of them."

Emotional Maladjustment and Personality Disorders

Numerous researchers have investigated the emotional adjustment of children and the families of children with articulatory disorders, and most have concluded that there is a considerable amount of maladjustment among parents of children with articulation disorders. Sometimes, the emotional reactions of parents toward their child's poor speech appear to have an adverse effect on the child's speech. Often, the articulation problem exists in children who experience certain unusual home situations such as a disturbed home membership where both parents work or are away for long periods of time. Speech clinicians have often used parent counseling along with therapy in many cases, finding it a helpful adjunct to therapy. *Warning*: Don't overgeneralize from such studies; don't jump to conclusions. Findings are drawn from many individuals and do not mean that any given case can be expected to follow the norm. We should, however, be alert to the possibility of some personality problems. After all, speech helps us adjust to our environment. The absence of acceptable speech is disturbing to the whole person, and it is impossible to separate cause and effect in much of the personality study.

Factors Related to Articulation Proficiency

Articulatory proficiency is dependent on a number of factors and must be judged within the context of such factors as age, intelligence, and educational achievement. In addition, anxiety and frustration may contribute to the problem and discouragement may serve to maintain it.

Age

The acquisition of sounds has been studied by numerous researchers to determine at what age children acquire certain sounds. Although there is some variation in the reported scales, there is also basic agreement. Even without the use of developmental articulation scales, we interpret articulation in terms of the speaker's age. The omissions that we accept in a three-year-old's speech would be highly unacceptable in the speech of a thirteen-year-old. Although you cannot go by a clock or calendar in determining when a child will acquire a specific sound, certain "rules of thumb" may serve as guidelines. We expect a two-year-old to be talking so that people outside the immediate family can understand at least 25 percent of what he is saying. We expect a six-year-old's speech to be 100 percent intelligible but not necessarily free from misarticulations. That is, he may still have faulty articulation but you can understand everything that he says. We expect an eight-year-old to have learned to articulate all of his sounds.

We accept certain misarticulations from certain age groups and not from others. A first grader who has not learned to articulate a *b* or *m* sound would be considered to have an articulation problem, but a first grader misarticulating an *r* or *ch* would not be considered to have abnormal articulation.

The following articulation scale is brief, but will give direction to your understanding of the order in which the sounds are learned. Many children learn to articulate most sounds at an earlier age than that given below. If, however, a child does not correctly articulate each sound by the specified age, he is considered to have defective articulation. Since vowel sounds come automatically, the following scale is only for consonant sounds.

A 3½-year-old child should correctly produce *p, b, m, h,* and *w.*

A 4½-year-old child should add to those the correct production of *t, d, n, k, g, ng,* and *y.*

A 5½-year-old child should add the correctly articulated *f.*

A 6½-year-old child should also produce the *v, sh, zh, l, s,* and voiced *th.*

A 7½-year-old child should also make the *ch, z, r, hw,* and the unvoiced *th.*

An 8-year-old child should have mastered the blends and have errorless articulation.

Intelligence

Most studies indicate some positive relationship between articulation and intelligence with the significant differences appearing at the lower measured IQ scores. Little differences are noted in children whose IQ scores exceed 70, but below that score a high correlation exists. This indicates that it does take a certain amount of intelligence to learn to articulate speech sounds, but that it does not require more than that possessed by the "slow learner." Intelligence, then, is a poor predictor of articulation ability except for the mentally retarded population. Too often the wrong conclusions are drawn. Too often it is assumed that because a child doesn't speak well he is mentally retarded. If we consider the verbal nature of most intelligence tests, we realize that poor speech may be reflected in lower IQ scores.

Educational Achievement

A number of studies have been conducted investigating the relationship between articulation and reading, articulation and spelling, and articulation and academic achievement. The majority of the studies concerned with reading ability have indicated a positive relationship between reading and articulatory proficiency. Studies by Yedinak (31), Everhart (32), FitzSimons (33), and Weaver (34), all found the group with articulation errors to be lower in reading scores than those without articulation defects. Studies concerned with the effect of speech training on reading ability indicate that reading scores are raised when children receive speech training (35). Furthermore, considerable evidence indicates that children with articulation errors tend to have more spelling errors (21) and that instruction in speech improvement results in improved spelling ability (36).

With the reported relationship between articulation errors and academic skills of reading and spelling, it is not surprising that there is also a relationship between articulation and academic achievement. Nelson (37) reported that a group of school children with articulation defects averaged one letter grade lower than their more articulate classmates in their academic achievement. He also found that seventh-grade children with defective articulation received lower marks on language, reading, and work habits. Winitz suggests that "articulation correction should be the first 'course' for those children with articulatory errors" (29). Indications are strong that the entire educational experience would be greatly enhanced by such remediation. Often, however, primary-grade children are not included in speech correction programs, since maturation alone corrects many misarticulations. The problem here is concerned with what happens to the "whole child" while we wait to see if he will outgrow his problem.

Anxiety and Frustration

Some factors serve to maintain and aggravate the speech problem. Anxiety and frustration in speech situations tend to increase as the child gets older. His speech errors become more noticeable as he enlarges his peer world with different and more playmates. Parents tend to become more concerned as the child matures. He may be corrected over and over by his parents, teased by other children, and made to feel a failure in many ways. Parents begin to suspect what neighbors have already decided—that the child is mentally retarded. Frustration builds up and adds to the difficulty in speaking situations, for it makes speech harder. The child learns that each time he opens his mouth he will somehow be hurt, but he does not learn to correct his error.

Discouragement

Many children with articulation errors learn to cover up their problem. They learn to mumble so that the listener is unable to detect misarticulations. They may learn certain undesirable behaviors that will tend to make them excluded rather than included in the group, or they may learn to be the "seen but not heard child," thus avoiding the necessity for speech. Being constantly corrected by people who do not know remedial procedures does not correct the problem. Furthermore, it is discouraging to the child always to be admonished to try harder but never to succeed.

Evaluation

A speaker's speech is evaluated by the listener. It may be pleasing, efficient, and communicative, or it may be unpleasant to listen to or not readily understood. If a child in your classroom has speech characterized by misarticulations, you may make the above-described type of evaluation—that is, he doesn't speak plainly. On the other hand, you may want more specific information about his articulation, and the way you gain this is through testing. Articulation tests come in a variety of forms from very simple screenings to extremely complicated deep testing of a variety of articulatory skills.

If there is a speech clinician in the school system, he may screen the speech of all children; he may screen the speech of only selected grades; or he may rely on teacher referrals for identification of articulation disorders. If there is no speech clinician, the classroom teacher may at times want to do some articulation screening. Research indicates that classroom teachers are efficient in simple articulation testing with a minimum of instruction (38). Basically, articulation tests may be divided into three kinds: (a) screening tests, (b) diagnostic tests, and (c) deep tests. Ordinarily the classroom teacher would not perform these, but it would he helpful for him to be familiar with the kinds of testing that may be done.

Screening involves testing a few of the more important sounds for the purpose of identifying problems, not analyzing them. Such tests may sample only frequently misarticulated sounds such as *s*, *l*, *r*, *th*, *v*, and *f*. The procedure may involve showing the child a picture and letting him tell you what it is. It may involve your saying the word and having the child repeat the word. Some screening tests are done by showing the child an object and saying, "What is this?" Some are constructed so that the child supplies the missing words, for example, "You comb your____[hair]." With some screenings you engage the child in conversation by asking simple questions or you may show him an action picture and ask him to tell you what is happening in the picture. For those who can read well, the screening may involve having the child read a specially prepared paragraph of selected sentences.

The more informally constructed or open-ended the test, the more difficult it is to identify accurately the error sounds. It is easier to listen for only one sound at a time than to identify errors in connected speech. Having the child engage in conversation, however, yields a more valid sample of his usual articulation of sounds. Some screenings may be performed by the classroom teacher if no speech clinician is available.

Diagnostic tests are designed to test all sounds and blends. They are used as follow-up tests to the screening. After a child has been identified by a screening test as having an articulation problem, the specific sounds that he misarticulates and in what contexts must be determined. These are important considerations in determining the severity of the problem, the prognosis for correction, and the therapy indicated. It is doubtful that a classroom teacher would administer diagnostic articulation tests.

Deep tests are designed to test one sound in all contexts. We do not always articulate a given phoneme (sound) in exactly the same manner. The sounds that come before it and after it color our production of a phoneme. Often the speech clinician needs information obtained from deep testing in attempting to determine prognosis for correction and in planning therapy. The classroom teacher would not do deep testing.

Stimulability testing has prognostic value. This involves instructing the child who misarticulates a sound to watch the teacher or clinician articulate the word and then to produce the word himself. If the child can correct his error through this imitation, the indication is that prognosis for articulation correction is better than if he is unable to do so with the help of the model. Having a child say a nonsense syllable containing the error sound is also used to determine if he can correctly hear and produce the sound in question. The more stimulable the child is, the easier it will probably be for him to correct his error. Classroom teachers may use this procedure in their screening.

Word lists containing the consonant sounds in a somewhat developmental sequence (beginning with easier or earlier learned sounds) may be helpful to a regular classroom teacher who wishes to test a child's speech for specific error sounds. The following list may be used as suggestions for pictures, objects, or words to illustrate each sound.

phoneme	
p	*p*ie, *p*ig, *p*encil, a*pp*le, *pupp*y, cu*p*, ca*p*
b	*b*ox, *b*u*bb*le, *b*oot, *b*a*b*y, tu*b*, ta*b*le, ro*b*e
t	*t*able, *t*oes, ki*tt*y, bo*tt*le, ha*t*, co*t*
d	*d*uck, *d*ig, *d*oll, can*d*y, In*d*ian, be*d*
k	*c*up, *c*at, *c*ookie, ba*c*on, *c*ake, boo*k*
g	*g*un, *g*oose, wa*g*on, ti*g*er, e*gg*, le*g*
f	*f*ish, *f*inger, *f*arm, tele*ph*one, lea*f*, mu*ff*
v	*v*alentine, *v*acuum, se*v*en, ele*v*en, sto*v*e
~~th~~ (voiceless)	*th*umb, *th*imble, bir*th*day cake, mou*th*, tee*th*
th (voiced)	fea*th*er, fa*th*er, mo*th*er, bro*th*er, wea*th*er
s	*s*aw, *s*oap, bi*c*ycle, poli*c*eman, mou*s*e, hou*s*e
z	*z*ebra, *z*oo, *z*ipper, no*s*e, eye*s*
sh	*sh*oe, *sh*eep, wa*sh*ing, di*sh*es, o*c*ean, fi*sh*, pu*sh*
zh	plea*s*ure, televi*s*ion (not necessary to test; if *sh* is defective, *zh* will probably be also)
ch	*ch*air, *ch*icken, *ch*in, pit*ch*er, wat*ch*, mat*ch*
j	*j*ump, *j*ello, sol*d*ier, en*g*ine, bri*dg*e
m	*m*onkey, *m*an, ca*m*el, ca*m*era, ha*mm*er, co*m*b, ha*m*
n	*kn*ife, *n*est, *n*ose, ru*nn*ing, ba*n*a*n*a, su*n*, gu*n*
ng	swi*ng*, dri*n*k, ha*ng*er, fi*ng*er, ri*ng*
l	*l*amp, *l*ion, ba*ll*oon, ye*ll*ow, ba*ll*
r	*r*abbit, *r*adio, fa*r*m, ca*r*, sta*r*
y	*y*arn, *y*ellow, on*i*on
w	*w*indow, *w*agon, *w*atch, spider-*w*eb, bo*w*-bow
h	*h*ouse, *h*at, *h*orse, *h*and
wh	*wh*eel, *wh*ite, *wh*istle, pin *wh*eel

NOTE: Not all sounds are spelled with the letter representing the phoneme. For instance, the *k* sound is often spelled *c*; likewise the *c* may represent the *s* sound. Although "onion" does not contain the letter *y*, it does contain the *y* sound, and the same is true for the *ng* sound in "drink."

Therapy

Isolating and correcting defective speech sounds can be considered the goal of articulation therapy. The many different approaches to articulation therapy are evidence of different rationales and techniques, yet they actually have a great deal in common. Many of the earlier therapies relied heavily on instructing the client concerning the management of his articulators or on the clinician's manipulating the client's articulators. Some therapies have relied heavily on ear training (teaching the client to identify the target sound and discriminate between it and other sounds). Some therapies incorporate procedures aimed at heightening the client's awareness of the movement of his articulators. Some advocate working on the correction of only one sound at a time; some suggest a multi-phonemic approach. Some advocate individual therapy only, some group therapy, and some a combination.

The reader can readily see that clinicians may vary in their articulation therapy approaches; yet, they will probably all incorporate certain similarities. They will all probably begin with some form of making the client aware of his error. Most will use some form of progressive approximation (aiding the client in coming closer and closer to the accepted articulation of the error sound). Most clinicians will present a model of the correct sound and the client attempts to reproduce it. Most therapies begin production of the target sound by having the client produce the correct sound in small utterances (in isolation, syllables, or words). Some form of behavior modification is the rule. This may vary from unsystematically rewarding correct responses with verbal praise, gold stars, prizes, etc., to a highly structured program of operant conditioning.

The Role of the Classroom Teacher

The classroom teacher has two functions: (a) support and reinforce the work of the school speech clinician and (b) provide speech improvement for all children. The speech-improvement program should include articulation training.

Although there are many approaches to therapy that the speech clinic may employ, the classroom teacher's instruction is concerned with improving the articulatory skills of all the children in the classroom. Certain therapy principles have been found to be successfully used by classroom teachers in their speech-improvement lessons.

Formerly, many speech clinicians have spent a great deal of articulation therapy time in what is called ear training. This consists of teaching the child to identify his error sound and to discriminate it from other sounds. Recent studies tend to indicate that individual therapy time can more profitably be spent beginning with teaching the child to produce the error sound. In speech improvement, however, where the teacher is dealing with an entire class, there appears to be merit in introducing the sound in a different way. The method that has proved successful with many speech-improvement teachers is described below.

First (a) identify the sound being presented. Give it a name or a personality. The *p* sound could be the "popcorn" sound, the *f* the "angry kitty" sound, the *sh* the "be quiet" sound, the *s* the "Sammy Snake" sound, etc. (b) Present the sound in isolation. Obviously, you do not expect children to have much opportunity in normal conversation to hear or use an isolated speech sound, but it may help to strengthen identification of the sound when it can be heard alone—not lost in a host of other sounds. This can be done using classroom activities in which children respond when they hear "their sound." There are many forms of quiet responses that may be made, such as holding up a picture representing their sound or giving a certain signal to indicate recognition. After the children are able to recognize the sound, have them discriminate the sound from other sounds—first gross differences such as *g* and *p*, then finer discriminations such as *f* and *p*. Young children may have to be taught the concept of "same and different" or "alike and different" in order to show discrimination.

Following the ear training with the isolated sound, (c) add a vowel to the sound. Use vowels that are different in appearance and sound such as the *ah*, *ee*, and *oo*. Next, have the children (d) discriminate nonsense syllables containing the sound being taught from other sounds, as *pah* from *kah*, and *pee* from *fee*. When he can do this, (e) move on to the same kind of discrimination in words and then in phrases. Games involving the speech sounds will motivate the learning process.

Following the auditory training period, speech-improvement lessons should (f) provide opportunities for children to produce the target sound beginning with isolation, syllables, words, and phrases. One word of caution: children may "over-articulate" a sound when producing it in isolation, so it may not be a good idea to spend undue time on this. Pairing the sound with a vowel should eliminate the distortion that over-articulating may create, and the teacher may choose to omit production in isolation. On the other hand, this simple step may be accomplished in a short time and may constitute a helpful preliminary to subsequent production steps.

The final step is (g) carry-over, or conversation. For most of the children, the speech-improvement work will have served only to refine their speech skills. For children with minor defective articulation, however, such work may well provide the necessary remediation instruction. For the more severe cases it may well facilitate the work of the school speech clinician.

The child who is in therapy will benefit from a classroom teacher who works closely with the speech clinician. For instance, the carry-over phase is not only generally the most difficult part of therapy but it is also the most important. It is often best early in the production phase to select a few words in which the child can produce the error sound correctly and call these by some special name such as "our words" or your "good speech words." The child should understand that he is never to misarticulate these words. If he does, he should immediately correct himself. To do this he needs help. The speech clinician will often enlist the assistance of the child's mother or of his teacher in helping monitor his articulation of these few words. Teachers, too, may use this procedure with their speech-improvement programs. Whenever one of these special words is heard produced correctly, a non-verbal signal can be used to say to the child "well done." This can be a smile, a special signal such as a finger in the air or touching your chin. Likewise, if the child is heard to misarticulate the sound, a prearranged signal should be used to say non-verbally to the child that he has slipped up. A pencil stuck in the teacher's hair, or a tug at the earlobe could serve the purpose. The goal is to bring the error to the child's conscious level without constant correction or nagging and without interrupting his speech.

Follow the use of a few key words with setting up a specific time each day for the child to be speech conscious and to use the new sound. This could be during a certain meal each day, during one hour of the day, during one class recitation each day, etc. At any rate, the carry-over phase of the correction of the sound is extended to all words used during that period. The same kind of monitoring assistance that was used with the key words can be used here. Eventually, the carry-over should filter out into the remainder of the child's day until his error sound is no longer incorrectly used in his speech. The carry-over aspect of articulation therapy is usually the most difficult, but it is also the most important.

If a speech correctionist is available, he or she and the teacher must form a team whose objective is the best speech that the individual speech-defective child can achieve. Correctionist and teacher will remember that the child is a complete personality and that at no time can his speech problem be divorced from his problems as an individual. The teacher is in a position to help in many ways other than in the teaching of a specific sound. For instance, if the child is scheduled for speech therapy at a particular time, it can be very helpful to him and to the therapist to aid in his keeping his appointment. In a group of twenty-five or thirty children, if the point is made that all can aid in remembering, usually someone will remember. A simple notice in the corner of a chalkboard such as "Jimmy, 1:15" to be left unerased will probably result in someone in the room remembering to help remind Jimmy without disturbing the rest of the class.

If no speech correctionist is available, the teacher may be able to improve the articulatory skills of the children in his or her class through a speech-improvement program along the lines described above. In order to teach speech sounds, however, you must understand the sounds of the language. Refer to the presentation of the sounds in Chapter 2. Check this list for your understanding of English speech sounds and then write some familiar words and phrases, using sound symbols rather than spelling with letters. Check your transcriptions with a dictionary.

It is important for the classroom teacher to remember that maturation alone does correct many articulation errors; however, we have no way of knowing for certain if this will happen in a given case. Training in hearing the sounds, discriminating between sounds, and using the sounds correctly will all speed the process of articulation maturation. It can, therefore, be reasoned that time spent in this part of the language program is profitable, since (a) for the children who may not otherwise correct all of their errors, the correction is a great benefit and (b) for those who would otherwise "outgrow" their misarticulations, the instruction hastens the process. Speech improvement is a vital part of any school curriculum. It should be viewed so by both teacher and students. If it is done haphazardly and only when thought of, it may not be done well. It should be planned, scheduled, and presented in a developmental sequence. If a time is set aside for speech improvement, then it is given the status of any other area of instruction both to the students and to the teacher. More specifically, speech improvement should be an important part of the language program.

General Suggestions for the Classroom Teacher

1. The classroom teacher will be able to help the speech clinician by acquainting him with the child's response to classroom and play situations.
2. He will also be able to tell the speech clinician much about the child's home and family situations.
3. The teacher needs a basic understanding of how sounds and their symbols function in the English language.
4. It will help if the teacher has a reasonably pleasant voice and good articulation himself.
5. The teacher will help the child by understanding his difficulties and by encouraging him in self-expression.
6. He should also help to reassure the child as to his importance as an individual.
7. He should encourage the child to participate in other activities where he will have a greater opportunity to be successful.

8. He must at all times remember that the child is a "complete personality" and not just a "case for speech correction."
9. He should assist all children in the classroom to learn and use clear, articulate speech.
10. He must make oral communication rewarding.

Chapter 4
Disordered Language Development

What does a teacher say to a mother who brings a non-verbal child to be entered in the first grade? What understandings does the teacher need in order to work effectively with a six-year-old who started talking only a year or two ago? Should a teacher attempt to correct the articulation of a child whose expressive language use is very limited? These and many other questions present themselves annually to kindergarten and primary grade teachers throughout the nation. What is the source of this kind of questioning?

For years the terms DELAYED SPEECH or DELAYED LANGUAGE have been used to describe the speech problem of such children, although authorities recognized that the disorder is not merely a problem of speech that is somewhat delayed in appearing—that it is a broader language disorder. In an effort to describe the problem more specifically, some authorities have recently adopted the terms DISORDERED LANGUAGE DEVELOPMENT, DEVIANT LANGUAGE, and LANGUAGE DEFICIENCY. The term probably most generally accepted is DELAYED LANGUAGE. We will use these terms interchangeably.

The puzzling problem of disordered language development (by whatever label given it) may be far more prevalent than many incidence studies indicate. The Mid-Century White House Conference Report placed the prevalence of delayed language at 0.3 percent (11), yet Wood (39) says that delayed language development occurs with greater frequency than other communication disorders and she gives the following explanation: (a) adults in this supersonic age tend to impose stricter demands on children for earlier and more accurate speech development; (b) more parents have become aware of developmental schedules and seek professional help earlier; (c) the mortality rate at birth has been reduced so that children suffering traumatic deliveries are now more likely to survive; and (d) specialists have become more skilled in the early detection of speech and language problems.

As previously noted, the development of speech progresses along certain relatively similar lines in the so-called average child, and marked deviations from this developmental pattern are viewed as disorders in speech development. The "average" child begins to talk during his second year, saying his first words around twelve months and phrases around eighteen months. This is viewed as his "speech readiness" period. Naturally, you cannot go strictly by developmental scales but must be guided by both the child's physiological and neurological maturity. Rate of maturation varies for the nervous system just as it does for the skeletal system and prohibits the establishment of rigid time restrictions for any developmental stage. Twenty-four months, however, has been established as the mean age for the development of speech that is intelligible to people outside the immediate family. In the absence of any evident cause for the failure to develop speech, any child who does not begin to speak intelligible two-word phrases by the time he is two years old should be referred to a speech pathologist. The longer speech is delayed, the more difficult it is to teach. The longer such children go without receiving help in attaining a normal means of communication, the more they tend to ignore the speech of others.

Characteristics

The difficulty encountered in placing disordered language development in any one symptomatic category has resulted in long listings of the various ways in which language may appear to be delayed. "There is usually a deficiency in vocabulary, a retardation in the development of conventional sentence structure, and often a marked inadequacy in the formulation of ideas. . . . The child just does not have the means of communication available" (39).

The problem is more than that of a severe articulation defect, since children with delayed language are also handicapped linguistically and semantically. Berry (40) describes the problem as one in which the manner or content of the child's language usage is significantly below the norm for children of his age. She includes the child who continues to rely almost entirely upon gestures when he should be using oral words; the physically normal child who uses oral words but in so mutilated and distorted a fashion that few people can understand him; the child whose vocabulary and sentence length and complexity vary significantly and undesirably from the quantitative norms for his age and sex. In addition, there are those who do not understand speech. These behavioral characteristics lead us to this definition: "delayed language is failure to understand or speak the language code of the community at a normal age" (2).

The average classroom teacher is not likely to encounter a child with a serious language disorder because the very nature of the child's disorder may result in his non-admission to school. His lack of language development often results in his being placed in a class for exceptional children—usually the mentally retarded. Sometimes such a child is placed in a class with normal children of a younger age group. For the most part, however, the delayed-language children encountered in the "normal" classroom will be those who have begun to talk but did so at a significantly later age or in a deviant manner.

Language disorders among school-age children may vary from a complete failure to use oral language, at one extreme, to an almost complete failure for a child to be understood despite evident strong efforts to communicate verbally, at the other extreme. In between these extremes, of course, lie the usual variations, including those with limited but readily intelligible vocabularies to those who have moderately large but only sometimes intelligible vocabularies. Often, the use of gestures supplements the speech in order to effect communication. Some children become quiet and withdrawn—the "seen not heard" children.

Many children who enter school with deviant language development are likely to present articulatory problems by the time they reach the second or third grade (12). They do not suddenly develop their articulatory difficulties, but rather their articulatory proficiency was disordered along with their language development. It was not until they began to manage language that the articulatory aspect of their overall development became more apparent. Children with severe oral linguistic impairment are not likely to advance beyond the primary grades because their disorder usually manifests itself in all areas of language. Exceptions, of course, exist, since some of them learn to read and write, but usually difficulties in these areas accompany difficulties in learning to speak.

Such children often need the assistance of the speech clinician to improve their articulation proficiency and sometimes such a professional is unavailable. In either case, the classroom teacher plays a key role in the language development of these children. For this reason, it appears realistic to endeavor to equip teachers with understandings concerning the causes, evaluation, and remediation for such children. This does not mean that the teachers will perform a differential diagnosis and initiate a therapy program, but rather that they will understand the problem and the procedures that would be beneficial as well as those procedures that would be detrimental.

Causes

Although the treatment of any disorder appears to be the important concern, sometimes the determination of the cause alters the treatment. Authorities emphasize both the importance of identifying the cause and also our frequent inability to do so.

. . . it is important that a careful and thorough study of the child's development and environment be made . . . in no other speech disorder it it so necessary to find and eliminate the cause, and the teacher should leave untapped no source of information which might lead to a knowledge of the origin of the child's lack of intelligible speech (3).

Yet, according to Wood (39), some causes are not known and others are not understood completely; at times more than one factor is reported as the cause; and available methods frequently are not inclusive enough or incisive enough to incorporate all of the many dimensions that should be considered in determining the degree of the problem.

The determination of causal factors in children with language disorders is a complex process. If a child is severely handicapped in his use of speech, probably no one test instrument can supply all of the information needed to classify the causal factors. The combined clinical judgments of specialists from various disciplines are needed. It should be pointed out that during clinical investigation of the causal factors, the development of language is not postponed. Usually therapy directed toward the development of language is initiated during the assessment period. Although, as already pointed out, the determination of the exact cause is often impossible, such a determination is needed to establish the educational objectives for the child. One wants to know if he is dealing with a deaf child, a mentally retarded child, or one who failed to develop speech because of environmental influences.

Causes may be classified in a number of ways, but it is appropriate to consider them as (a) organic deficiencies and disorders, (b) environmental causes, and (c) emotional disturbances in the child.

Organic Deficiencies and Disorders

Mental Retardation

This is the most common cause of language deficiency. In fact, "delayed language development is a predominant characteristic" (2) of the mentally retarded, with the severely retarded never acquiring speech. Below the mental age of five years, speech acquisition correlates roughly with the amount of retardation. Sometimes a language problem is the cause of apparent low intelligence. Examples have been cited of delayed language children whose IQ scores rose from ten to thirty points following the development of language (39). Language deficiency may be a very simple yardstick for measuring mental retardation, but it can also be a very inaccurate one.

Hearing Impairment

Another important cause of difficulty in developing language is impaired hearing. Since the language code is learned from the environment, the deaf child has little way of acquiring this normally, and it is generally understood that deafness results in speechlessness unless the child receives special teaching. What is not so well known is that the child with only impaired hearing may also suffer in his language acquisition. He may have enough hearing for him to appear to respond to sound normally, yet not enough for him to learn adequate speech. Many of these children, both the deaf and the hearing impaired, go undiagnosed until their failure to learn to talk causes the family to seek help. Usually parents are concerned when their child doesn't begin to talk by roughly age two or three, but for a number of reasons they may postpone seeking professional help. Advice from neighbors and family that "he will talk when he is ready," uncertainty about where to seek professional help and lack of awareness of the significance of the language delay may all contribute to this. Some parents wait until the child is approaching school age, when the child's language acquisition suddenly becomes an urgent concern, resulting in their seeking professional help.

There are children who appear to be able to hear and respond appropriately to non-speech sounds, and nevertheless fail to develop speech (40). Sound discrimination is important to the successful imitation of sounds. Unlike sensations such as taste, pressure, or pain in which there can be great individual variability, sound discrimination must be greatly alike for all people interpreting it. Some children appear to be unable to make the fine discriminations required for intelligible speech. Some appear to have a short auditory memory span and their attempts to reproduce connected speech may result only in "verbal hash."

Other Organic Causes

Brain injury, even mild cerebral dysfunction, affects a child's ability to perceive, store, and retrieve sequential stimuli (2), thus impairing his language acquisition. When brain injury occurs prior to the learning of speech, the condition may not be suspected until the child fails to talk at the expected age. These are often puzzling children and difficult to teach. They often have perceptual difficulties and fail to develop laterality. They have a short attention span and are unpredictable in behavior. The language learning that they are able to accomplish does not follow normal steps of language learning. It is unlikely that the severely affected child will be in the regular classroom, but he may be placed in the special education class, frequently misdiagnosed.

The child with minimal brain damage may be in the regular classroom, however, and his inconsistent behavior may well present puzzling problems for those who try to teach him. The classroom teacher's primary contribution may be in referring him for adequate diagnosis, in helping to locate appropriate speech therapy, and in trying to understand, as best he can, the confusion and apprehension that the child and his family experience.

Defective structures of the speech mechanism have long been listed as contributing factors to the failure to develop normal speech. The same can be said with reference to language acquisition as was said about articulation— these may well be considered only contributing factors rather than causes. Ill health is also traditionally thought of as a contributing factor. If a child's illness is of sufficient intensity and duration, it certainly could affect language acquisition adversely. "The capacity to learn language is of practical value only prior to puberty" (2) and a child who spends his prepubertal years just managing to survive may leave undeveloped his native capacity to learn language.

Environmental Causes

An environment unfavorable to the development of language can produce non-speaking or poorly speaking children. Although a child may be considered to have an innate language-learning ability, there are environmental conditions that may be detrimental to normal acquisition of language. Often such causes are so obscured that they are impossible to identify; others are so obvious that they virtually identify themselves. Often one cause alone is insufficient to retard language, but a combination of several unfavorable environmental influences may result in a failure to use speech.

Lack of Motivation

A child cannot be expected to speak unless there is some reason for him to want to speak. If his speech efforts are ignored, then there is little reward and hence no motivation to continue this activity. More frequently, however, the child lacking motivation may be the overprotected child. "Some mothers become so skillful at anticipating their child's every wish that the performance astounds the bystander. This appalling situation arises especially when the child is an only child or has been ill a great deal or is handicapped in some way" (3). The child may, for this or some other reason, fail to experience a need to change from his infantile, prelingual way of getting responses from, and responding to, his environment to the more conventionalized and mature way of accomplishing his ends (40). If his pantomine and assortment of grunts and groans are adequate, then wherein lies the motivation to change his behavior?

A Silent Environment

Silence does not provide a child with the kind of experience that he needs to acquire speech. Cases have been cited in which a child was raised by deaf mutes and did not acquire speech. Other less dramatic examples occur in situations where little speech is carried on in the home for a number of individual reasons or in cases of parental absenteeism. The author evaluated a two-and-one-half-year-year-old non-speaking boy whose mother had recently been hospitalized with a severe psychotic condition. The case history revealed that this only child, whose father was studying toward an advanced graduate degree, had spent his entire life with a mother who had not talked since the birth of the baby. With the exception of the absolutely necessary activity involved with caring for an infant, she spent her time reading. This had been the only environment the child had ever known—a silent one. The importance of a speaking environment to the acquisition of speech is apparent.

Poor Teaching Techniques

In spite of the lack of common knowledge among parents concerning teaching a baby to talk, most children do quite well. Some, however, fail to acquire speech simply because of the poor teaching techniques used with them. Knowing little about the acquisition of speech, most parents expect the miracle to happen but usually attempt to speed up the onset by bombarding the child with stimulation by the time he is a month or so old. This is fine, but some either give up or lose interest before the baby is old enough to profit maximally from such stimulation. Still others, believing that baby talk is undesirable, provide stimulation through such complicated words as "bicycle," "mother," and "refrigerator," and may rebuke the baby's efforts to say "ball" when he produces the approximation "ba".

Happily, most parents instinctively reinforce the child's early attempts by imitating them, and after the child has learned a few words of his own choosing, they seem to know how to go on to teaching a new word made up of sounds that the child enjoys or can approximate. Sometimes, however, the happy accidents do not occur to provide the child the maximum in good teaching techniques.

Influence of Siblings

Some studies indicate that children who arrive in a family in which there are already children to provide them with poor speech models may have some language-learning difficulty. There are also the psychological problems of sibling rivalry. This is frequently encountered in the case of the birth of a new sibling. "The new baby, a crying, non-talking child, literally steals the show from the older child. The latter, in the hope of winning back some of the lost attention and what he believes to be lost affection, may emulate and imitate the ways of the 'usurper'" (40). Unwitting parents add to this problem when they try to motivate more maturity by saying that "only babies" behave in certain ways, for example, cry, wet their pants, drink from a bottle. For the child who is competing with the baby, this suggests further ways for him to cope with his rival.

Twins create a special environmental influence that seems to be disadvantageous for speech learning and language development. Twins not only begin to speak later than do single children, their language tends to remain significantly deficient until after they enter school (41). They often develop special words or private language (idioglossia) or gestures with which they communicate with each other but which are not understood by other people.

Bilingualism

Having two languages spoken in the home may create a language barrier for some children. Some parents deliberately attempt to teach their children two languages at the same time, but usually the bilingual environment occurs when one generation or part of the family speaks a foreign language and the younger members or other part of the household speak English (or the language of the country in which they live). Such confusion may result in language retardation (3). Research shows that children learning only one language develop vocabularies in excess of those learning two languages even when the two languages are added (40). For most bilingual children there appears to be no significant problem created; however, if a child is experiencing some difficulty in acquiring speech, bilingualism is an area of concern. In such cases the confusion of two languages should be eliminated until the child is well established in one language.

Psychological or Emotional Disturbances

A child's failure to acquire normal language may reflect an emotional disturbance. This may be a severe psychotic condition, or it may be a relatively mild expression of insecurity or jealousy. Children with language disorders often appear to be excessively emotional children. Certainly, without adequate and commonly accepted means of adjustment, anyone is likely to be frustrated. Children with a language disorder, lacking the most common of all means of adjustment to the environment, speech, tend to develop into frustrated, overly emotional individuals. Some lack only the expressive language with which to make their thoughts and wishes known; other may lack the inner language with which to "think" through their adjustments. It is easily understood that these children frequently resort to temper displays when their efforts to communicate are not understood. Excessive and continued dependence on a few persons, usually their family, for the satisfaction of their needs, prevents them from gaining a proper degree of independence as they mature. Many of them cling excessively to their parents, thus adding to their problem of maturing. Sometimes the child's history reveals that his language delay is only one aspect of a picture of general emotional immaturity. Such cases may occur in the instance of extreme sibling rivalry.

Negativism

Most two-year-olds go through a period when "NO" appears to be their only word, but an attitude of extreme negativism may be responsible for interference in normal speech development. This attitude may be a general characteristic of the child's behavior or it may be directed toward particular persons responsible for his speech training, such as his parents or his teacher. It is not always possible to trace the emotional disturbances to a person or persons, but the attitude of "I won't talk because you want me to!" is exhibited. Unwitting parents and speech pathologists as well frequently reward the very behavior that they wish to extinguish by giving the child much attention focused on his refusal to talk. Finding a way to make speech appear rewarding to the child and to make silence unrewarding or even punishing to him usually results in his voluntary abdication of mutism. Often it is extremely difficult for us to identify the things that we are doing to reward speechlessness in the negative child and we may need to enlist the aid of an observer to help do this. Furthermore, we make erroneous assumptions about what is rewarding and punishing. The child may be gaining more attention from his failure to talk than he would from conforming to our expectation. If attention is his goal, then we may well be rewarding his mutism with our bribery to talk.

Autism

This is one of the most severe forms of emotional disturbance resulting in a language disorder. In the most extreme form of withdrawal or detachment from the environment, the child may seem unable to hear and may be diagnosed as having peripheral deafness. Such children show little response to sounds—especially human sounds, although they may be observed improvising and playing with sounds. The classroom teacher seldom encounters autistic children in the regular classroom, but they may be found, usually misdiagnosed, in classes for the mentally retarded or for the deaf and hard-of-hearing. The classroom teacher, however, cannot assume that he will never encounter an autistic child. The author evaluated one such child whose parents, refusing to accept the diagnosis, had moved her from one school to another, always registering her in a normal classroom. As soon as her problem was diagnosed, they would move to another town and repeat the procedure. A number of regular classroom teachers came in contact with this autistic child.

Multiple Causes

Many of the listed causes are found individually in many normally speaking children. This is one of the reasons that identifying the cause of a language disorder in children is often difficult. Children often experience a number of possible causes, each individually insufficient to cause a language problem, but collectively constituting a significant barrier to language acquisition.

Evaluation

"Parents are usually concerned about their children if they are not following oral directions at least by two years of age or if they are not talking by the time they are three" (42). This concern often leads them to seek help that eventually takes them to a speech and hearing clinic for evaluation and therapy. In the case of the child without speech, the evaluation presents one of the clinician's most challenging tasks.

Van Riper (3) suggests that in order to understand the problem with which he is confronted, the clinician must first find out the extent of the disability. To do this the child must be placed in a situation where the need to communicate is very strong, and yet, one in which the child's security is not threatened. This, however, is not always an easy task to accomplish, but it is necessary for the clinician to be able to describe the child's language. Wood (39) points out that (a) the evaluation of language requires a multi-professional approach including medical, psychological, audiological, and speech and language evaluations; (b) test items used to evaluate language development may be lifted from larger test batteries; therefore, scores must be considered inferential and experimental; and (c) language evaluations generally are not designed to provide the examiner with absolute scores as much as they attempt to tap the child's areas of abilities and his weaknesses.

Information about the child's speech and the reasons explaining it must be sought. In general, information about the child's communication problem is obtained from three sources: (a) case history, (b) observations of the child's and parents' behaviors; and (c) evaluations of the child's responses on specific tasks or in specific test situations (1). All of this information must be integrated to form a single profile of the child and his speech.

The Case History

The case history may prove to be a valuable diagnostic instrument, since frequently much needed information can be obtained only from someone who knows the child, the conditions surrounding his birth and development, and other factors in his environment.

Observation

Careful and intelligent observation of the child's behavior can also be extremely helpful in understanding the child and his language development.

Since delayed language may be the common denominator for the deaf child, the brain-injured child, the emotionally disturbed child, and the mentally retarded child, awareness of the behavioral characteristics of each classification may aid the observer in noting significant behaviors. Myklebust (26) summarizes these descriptions as follows.

Children who are profoundly hard-of-hearing or deaf display laughter that is deficient in extent and spontaneity and reduced in tonal pattern and intensity variations. Smiling is used less frequently and less meaningfully than for normal expression. Crying is normal in amount and purpose. They are unusually sensitive to movement and other visual cues, perhaps appearing more alert because they notice things that normal children fail to notice. They are not different from normal children in development of motor skills, but may seem hyperactive, although such activity is purposeful. Perhaps, because they do not hear the noise they make, they may shuffle when they walk. Their social perception is not seriously impaired, but they may remain on the periphery of social situations, withdrawing somewhat and engaging themselves with objects, but not with the compulsive manner seen in emotionally disturbed children.

Brain-injured children laugh, smile, and cry but typically without intensity of feeling, the cry being typically a whine. They are not unduly sensitive to visual or tactile sensation. They may even ignore other sensory stimulation when involved in an activity. Unlike severely emotionally disturbed children, they do not ignore other persons. They do not seem to use facial expression effectively for communication. Their motor coordination is often inferior in walking, throwing, and kicking. Motor activity may be random and less persistent than in normal children. Frequently, there is hyperactivity that is compulsive in nature rather than deliberate and goal directed. Social perception is often impaired, the child making little distinction between friends and strangers, engaging poorly in play and being unsure of situations.

Severely emotionally disturbed children have abnormal patterns of laughing, smiling, and crying, depending upon the severity of their disturbance. Some children do not display these behaviors at all. They are not usually sensitive to tactile cues or to movement or other visual cues, and they are inattentive to the facial expression of others. In fact, a distinctive characteristic of autistic children is their refusal to look at the faces of others. They are usually healthy, well developed physically, and well coordinated. These children show a high degree of social imperception, disregarding the wishes of others, usually behaving as though others do not exist.

Mentally retarded children are like normal children in laughing, smiling, and crying, except that low-grade mentally defective children may not laugh and are unresponsive socially. They lack normal curiosity and are not unusually sensitive to visual or tactile sensations. Mentally retarded children are responsive to facial expression and to expressions of acceptance and warmth. Retardation in development of motor skills is characteristic of these children. While they may not ignore others, they may be slow in reacting to them. A lack of comprehension of the meaning of social situations is typical. Although they show emotional expression, it is typically in a manner immature for their chronological age.

Testing

Finally, some form of testing is needed to assess the child and his language. Present standardized intelligence tests, by themselves, cannot give a completely valid measurement of the mental-age level of children with severe language delay. Nevertheless, they serve as a valuable inferential tool. The child's hearing should also be tested. Finally,

Three basic types of linguistic abilities should be examined: vocabulary, grammar, and the functional use of language. . . . A test of vocabulary is a test of semantic ability. . . . A test of grammar is a test of one's knowledge of how language works. . . . [and] A test of the functional use of language . . . examines pragmatically how speech is used for communicative purposes (2).

The objectives, then, of the language evaluation are: (a) to determine if the child actually has a language problem, (b) to determine the nature and severity of the problem, (c) to determine the prognosis, and (4) to determine appropriate remedial procedures.

Therapy

Remediation procedures for language-impaired children may vary markedly because of the therapy approaches taken by clinicians, the severity and nature of the impairment, and the unique factors involved with individual children. Specific therapeutic procedures, therefore, are not dealt with in this brief discussion, but certain principles of therapy are applicable.

Early Intervention Is Important

The child who develops language normally will be constructing fully developed, grammatically accurate sentences by the time he is four years old; therefore, postponing therapeutic intervention with the language-impaired child removes him further from the age at which language acquisition is a natural phenomenon. In the case of mentally retarded children whose total development is retarded, direct therapy may be postponed somewhat until they reach a mental age sufficient for language acquisition. (This does not preclude parental guidance directed by the speech clinician.) Therapy may then be on-going until puberty, which sets the ceiling on speech acquisition. "If they progress as far as a mental age of 4 or 5, they should have reasonably normal language; if they reach a mental age of 2, they should have primitive rudiments of language; if below 2, they are likely to have almost none" (2).

Children whose language impairment is due to environmental influences usually make the most rapid progress in therapy if the environmental conditions can be improved. Likewise, those whose language disorder is associated with emotional conflicts often respond rapidly when the conflicts are resolved. Autistic children, however, usually present a picture of slow progress and require extended on-going therapy, as do the mentally retarded and neurologically impaired. Those with hearing impairment need early and continued therapy. In all cases, however, the principle of early intervention is important to optimum remediation.

The Terminal Goal of Therapy Is Normal Language

Pragmatically, this is not always a realistic goal. For instance, the severely mentally retarded may never acquire language. An accurate assessment, however, of the child and his language should enable the clinician to compare what the child does with what he should be able to do. Carefully chosen steps to move the child toward this goal then can be programed.

Therapy Procedures Generally Fit Roughly a Pattern of Operant Conditioning

Some procedures may be based primarily on trial and error for selection of steps and rewards. Others may be explicitly grounded on principles of learning and strictly follow principles of operant conditioning. From whichever theoretical position the clinician begins, steps involve finding (a) responses that can be systematically modified toward the desired terminal behavior and (b) the reinforcements that are rewarding to the individual child. The steps in the therapy program must be carefully selected to allow the child to move toward the terminal goal, just as the schedule of reinforcement is also important in the child's acquisition and retention of the desired behavior.

Two procedures that are frequently incorporated into therapy are (a) *imitation* and (b) *expansion*. For children with no demonstrable speech, teaching *imitation* may begin with non-verbal tasks, for instance, sitting in a chair, head movements, hand clapping, or placing objects in certain positions. For the child whose one-word responses consist of naming objects, imitation may involve teaching the use of the definite article by having the child imitate the clinician's model, for instance, "the man," "the ball," or "the car." Teaching verbs would follow the same procedure with such models as "The boy runs" or "The ball rolls." The progression in the imitation tasks must enable the child to gain the needed insight into how the language works and to acquire for himself the ability to use it functionally. The assumption underlying this therapy procedure is that the child will generalize from imitation to conversation—that enough practice in imitating the clinician's model of putting a noun and a verb together to make a rudimentary sentence will enable the child to do this in conversation. Many clinicians take a cue from parents' common teaching procedure involving *expansion* of the child's utterance. The child who reaches toward a flower and says, "Pretty" may have this repeated to him by his parents, as "See the pretty flower." This seems to be a natural teaching procedure for parents and it can be systematically incorporated into clinical management of language acquisition.

Parents and Teachers Are Often Involved in the Therapy Program

Although there is disagreement concerning the nature and extent of parental involvement, clinicians tend to rely on concerned people in the child's environment to carry out certain prescribed procedures. For the deaf child, it may be in the form of helping to teach him to look at the speaker or for the mentally retarded child, it may be to expand his primitive sentences. The list of examples may be endless, limited only by the imagination of the clinician and the limitations of the parent or teacher. Parents and teachers may also be involved in a program of reinforcement or reward for the child's use of the language structure being taught. Often programs of parent counseling are a part of the therapy procedure.

On-going Assessment of the Child and His Language Problem Is an Aspect of Therapy

Perhaps in no other disorder is it so imperative that the clinician maintain the function of evaluator. Goals may be altered; teaching methods may be changed; or hidden causes may emerge that have significance for clinical management. Furthermore, the child's expressive language delay may be only one aspect of a larger disorder involving several modalities, and careful observation of behaviors may give the clinician needed insights.

The Role of the Classroom Teacher

The emotional climate required for a child with a language problem should be understood by the clinician and the teacher and should be interpreted to the parents. First, *he needs to feel acceptance of his not talking*, regardless of the reasons associated with this failure in development; therefore, the teacher or clinician must react no differently to a child with little functional language, whether caused by a hearing deficit or serious emotional problem, than he would to any other child. The child will need acceptance and understanding of the kinds of compensatory skills that he may have already developed, and the teacher cannot force him to relinquish too soon such adjustive techniques as temper tantrums or furtive watching from the sidelines.

Second, *this child needs to feel respected for what abilities he has,* for what disabilities he struggles against. This does not mean praise, pity, or protection in disproportionate amounts, but faith in the child as a person able to cope with his own problems in ways suitable to his age, his maturation level, and the opportunities given him.

Third, *he needs to feel secure.* This requirement poses a particular problem for the teacher who is accustomed to being with children who are able to express their needs verbally. The problem will be further involved if the teacher himself does not feel secure with a silent child. The teacher must be imaginative, creative, and know many children well in order that he may infer when the silent child experiences fear, anxiety, frustration, and other feelings common to all children at times. The extent to which he can provide a reliable, consistent, organized environment with rational limits and the extent to which he can grant the child freedom to express and explore in his own way will also influence the security the child enjoys.

Fourth, *the child needs to feel that he belongs.* The problem of meeting this need may assume large proportions if the child who does not talk is with normally speaking children; yet, many children include the child with differences more readily and with less prejudice than do adults. The silent child will find ways other than verbal for participation. He may participate chiefly by just being there; he may watch what is going on and relive the experiences at home. It must be remembered, however, that the feeling of belonging is not just assumed by the adults. This child needs to share in what goes on—feeding the fish, washing the paint jars, putting away toys, passing the wastebasket. He needs to experience taking turns, waiting for the slower one, and sharing. All of these things help the child to feel a part of others' lives and to know that their lives include him. In short, "the need of the child with delayed language development to feel satisfaction and pleasure is not different from that of other children" (43).

It is perhaps easier to give the classroom teacher suggestions such as the above than it is to give specific suggestions, but somehow the teacher must give the child communicative experiences that will be rewarding. For example, an extremely shy child who does not talk in the classroom or one who is not yet talking would not want to be called on to tell an experience during sharing time; yet this child may get pleasure from a sharing experience that did not appear threatening to him. For instance, if such a child brought a toy to class, the teacher may ask the child if he will hold the toy before the class while the teacher tells about it. This allows the child to participate in the sharing without requiring him to communicate orally. Choral reading or speaking will give him further experience with communicating in a non-threatening situation. Later, this child may participate orally in small-group work and so on until he has had successful speaking experiences and time to develop more speech skills.

Children with disordered language development need to learn that speech is enjoyable before they become aware that with the acquisition of speech there is an assumption of communicative responsibility.

When pleasure replaces apprehension, goals for increased speech proficiency can be set. The child should be gently directed toward these goals about which incidentally, it is best that he have no conscious awareness at the outset of his school career. The teacher should, if possible, share information and objectives with the child's parents so that the proper attitudes may prevail in the home as well as in the school. (12)

In conclusion, "for a child to speak, he must have something to say, the need for saying it, security in the act of saying it and sufficient praise, encouragement and self-satisfaction to make the effort worthwhile" (44).

Chapter 5

Stuttering

Perhaps no other speech problem is viewed with so much apprehension, anxiety, bewilderment, and misunderstanding as the problem of stuttering. Volumes have been written regarding etiology and remediation; countless research studies have investigated the problem; thousands of dollars have been paid both to reputable clinics and to quacks as well for treatment; yet the stutterer stutters! This is not to say that no remediation has proved effective; rather that no consensus has emerged concerning cause and treatment, and that therapy failures persist side by side with therapy successes.

It is easier to describe stuttering behaviors than it is to define stuttering. Stuttering is characterized by abnormal rhythm in speaking. This may be in the form of a repetition of an initial sound or an entire word; it may be a prolongation of a sound; or the speaker may appear unable to emit a sound. Stuttering, therefore, appears to be a rhythm problem occurring when the flow of speech is interrupted abnormally by repetitions or prolongations of a sound, syllable, or posture, and/or by avoidance and struggle reaction (3). For the beginning stutterer, the non-fluencies or breaks in normal rhythm may be relatively free from tension and awareness; however, for the confirmed stutterer there may be not only definite awareness and anxiety, but also many accompanying mannerisms called secondary characteristics, or accessory features. Some of the more commonly observed secondary characteristics are facial grimaces, foot stamping, finger snapping, head shaking, and eye blinking. Therefore, not all of the abnormal behaviors are stuttering behaviors; some are coping behaviors that are associated with stuttering.

Stuttering has been defined as what the speaker does when trying not to stutter, or as an anticipatory, apprehensive, hypertonic, avoidance reaction analogous to a novice tightrope walker (13). He expects to fall off the rope (anticipatory); he dreads falling (apprehensive); he stiffens and becomes unsteady in anticipation of the fall (hypertonic); and, in trying to avoid falling, he overcorrects and falls (avoidance). The difficulty the walker experiences is in direct proportion to the amount of threat he perceives in the walking situation, just as the amount of disfluency the stutterer has is in direct proportion to the amount of threat he interprets the speaking situation to have. A very close look at stuttering behaviors alone (not coping behaviors) leads us to conclude that stuttering is the abnormal initiation of a sound. It is this abnormal initiation of the sound that results in the apparent repetitions and blocks.

Causes

Theories relative to the origin of stuttering behavior have varied widely—most with supportive research, but none with conclusive evidence. Basically, stuttering theories fall into one of three categories: (a) organic, (b) psychogenic, or (c) learned.

Some of the earliest explanations of the riddle of stuttering were *organically* based. Investigators have sought to discover relationships to muscle spasms, tongue abnormalities, central nervous system damage, metabolic processes, vitamin deficiencies, etc. Early theories have proved rather unpromising and many even absurd. Looking for the cause in the physiology of the individual became less popular during the middle part of this century, but recent theorists have begun to look further at organic factors. West (45) studied medical records of diabetics and epileptics with relation to the incidence of stuttering among the two groups. Finding no stutterers reported among diabetics and a higher than expected incidence among epileptics, he concluded that stuttering is a form of seizure called pyknolepsie. Eisenson (46) described stuttering as a form of perseverative behavior stemming from a neurological difference between stutterers and non-stutterers. Others have found differences in listening tasks, and some consider the problem to lie in a general neurological predisposition to stuttering. Webster (47) has theorized that a defective muscle insertion in the hearing mechanism causing defective auditory feedback is the cause of stuttering. He has programed instruction for remediation based on this theory and has reported therapy success in his laboratory.

Although the organic theorists place the origin of stuttering in the physiology, most of them suggest a learning component. They may suggest an organic weakness as a necessary component of stuttering, but that it must be triggered by emotional stress. Some feel that the organic component caused the original stuttering, but that the emotional reactions caused by it are responsible for maintaining the stuttering behaviors.

Stuttering as a manifestation of a *psychogenic* disturbance has also been investigated. Glauber, (48) one of the proponents of this explanation, based his theory on Freudian psychology and on the reports that Freud made in his writing on stuttering. Many psychologists and psychoanalyists have emphasized that stutterers are maladjusted persons. Coriat (49) wrote that stutterers are "infants who have compulsively retained the original equivalents of nursing and biting." Most of these theorists point to cases to support their views. It is difficult to evaluate this theory because it is difficult to determine whether the personality maladjustment causes the stuttering or is caused by the stuttering. The importance of learning is inherent in these theories, since they are based on the individual's learning through experiences to repress certain modes of behavior. These references to learning, like those of the organic theorists, are only in the broadest sense and do not explain the behaviors in terms of classical or instrumental conditioning.

Theories that stuttering is *learned* behavior have in some measure dominated much of the thinking and research for several decades. As already pointed out, both the organic and psychogenic theorists mention learning in their theories, but other theorists have described stuttering solely in terms of learning. Wendell Johnson, one of the most prolific researchers and writers concerning stuttering during the 1940s and 50s, was one of the chief proponents of the theory that stuttering is learned. His theory, however, is not in learning-theory terms. Johnson said that stuttering was born in the ear of the listener—that the stutterer becomes a stutterer after being so diagnosed. His is a semantic explanation often referred to as a semantogenic theory. For a concise and readable explanation of Johnson's views on stuttering, read *An Open Letter to the Mother of a Stuttering Child* (50). Other theorists, Brutten and Shoemaker (51) for example, have explained stuttering in learning-theory terms.

Basically, it is the contention of Johnson and others that fluency is a problem for all speakers, but particularly for the child who is just learning to talk—the child who has not learned to encode messages as quickly as we expect speech to flow. The child does a lot of stumbling and looking for the right word; he easily becomes excited and loses some of his acquired fluency. He needs practice in arranging words together in a fluent manner.

After all, rhythm appears to be the most important speech skill that the child between two and four years of age is acquiring. He is learning to become a speaker and his parents have come to think of him as a speaker. When he stumbles and falters, and parents react negatively to that stumbling and faltering, they may be inadvertently saying to him, "I am not pleased with you," "There is something wrong with you," or "You lack worth." Their admonishments to try harder usually achieve negative results. The child will try harder, all right, but pretty soon the fun will drop out of speaking and will be replaced with fear and apprehension about the speaking situation. Normal non-fluency then will become abnormal non-fluency.

We all know that extreme anxiety or fear may result in less fluency. The phrase, "frightened speechless," is not without meaning. We may have observed a normally fluent child caught in a fib, suddenly falter and stumble in his speech as he tries to explain his behavior—or we have seen a comedy situation on television or on stage where stuttered or non-fluent speech was used to convey to the audience that the comic is likewise caught in such a situation.

This, then, is a highly simplified version of Johnson's explanation of stuttering. We are all normally non-fluent. Children learning to use speech are especially so. Put abnormal pressure on us for fluent speech, and we tend to fall apart verbally. If our listeners label this stuttering and we think of speech as something difficult and of ourselves as stutterers, then we become just that. Our speech patterns of abnormal rhythm become habit patterns. The parents become anxious about hesitancies and repetitions, and the child, conscious of his parents' attitudes, begins to fear, avoid, or struggle to inhibit his speech hesitancies. The result is that it does appear that what he is doing to keep from stuttering is the very thing that causes the stuttering.

Learning theory, in general, states that stuttering is a learned behavior. According to this theory, stuttering has its origin in the early normal non-fluencies. Not all children display the same amount of verbal stumbling, just as not all display the same amount of other behaviors. Some of us are not verbal athletes, just as not all of us are physical athletes, but our self-concept affects our ability to use the skills we have most effectively. Not all children react to pressures in the same manner.

Perhaps there are *multiple causes*. Obviously, when there are so many conflicting views, not all can be exclusively correct. Perhaps the multiplicity of causes may allow each to be correct in certain instances or in certain combinations of circumstances. There could well be an underlying organic basis for stuttering that could be triggered by environmental influences. These environmental influences would not result in stuttering in a person not having the predisposition. For instance, if a predisposition to stuttering exists in a child, then emotional stress at an age when adequate speech function is precarious may result in a speech disturbance. It can likewise be reasoned that, in a child with pronounced genetic and neurologic predisposition to stuttering, the amount of emotional stress and anxiety needed to precipitate stuttering behavior may be minor; but for a child with minimal predisposition, a more severe emotional stress will be required. Once the involuntary repetitions of sounds and syllables have begun, the child soon learns to anticipate difficult sounds, words, and situations, and his stuttering behavior does become learned. More research is indicated before we have a definitive answer. In the meantime, the therapy approaches of people from each theoretical position often have many similarities.

Agreed-on "Facts" about Stuttering

With the volumes that have been written concerning what is not known or proved with regard to stuttering, perhaps it would be a good idea to look at some things that are known. Certain observed behaviors and collected research data give us some "agreed-on facts" regarding stuttering and the stutterer. Among these are:

1. The average stutterer stutters on only about 10 percent of his utterances. This means that 90 percent of the time he is fluent. Most stutterers will deny this, saying that they stutter on every word, and truly some do appear to do almost that. For the most part, however, they do not stutter as much as they think they do. This indicates that their stuttering is not as severe as they interpret it to be or that they overreact to their stuttering.

2. Most stutterings last only one or two seconds—or less. Again, most stutterers will deny this, saying that they get stuck for several minutes without being able to utter a sound or get stuck on a certain sound and repeat it for a longer period of time. Likewise, most listeners will also deny the short duration of blocks and repetitions reported by research. We are a verbal lot of people, and we fear silence. When the stutterer "gets stuck," the listener is uncomfortable because of the silence and tends to say the word for the stutterer if the word can be guessed. The stutterer is miserable because of the silence, but he doesn't appreciate having the word said for him. He may be embarrassed or angry about it. The struggle makes both the speaker and the listener uncomfortable; therefore, the time seems much longer than it actually is. Time always drags more during unpleasant experiences than during pleasant ones.

3. No two stutterers perform their stuttering in exactly the same way, and any one stutterer varies somewhat with time and can be trained to vary markedly. To say "He stutters" does not tell you the exact behavior that a person exhibits—it merely tells you that his speech has a rhythm disturbance. He may block for periods of time with no sound; or he may repeat a sound, syllable, word, or even phrase; or he may prolong a sound. He may seem relatively relaxed in doing so or extremely tense. He may have no accompanying gestures or secondary characteristics, or he may exhibit extreme facial grimaces or "starters." What a stutterer does as a beginning stutterer does not resemble what he does after becoming a confirmed stutterer, and, although he may be unable to stop stuttering, he can usually alter his stuttering behaviors—especially with training.

4. Stuttering begins, on the average, at about the age of three years—some earlier, some later. Remembering the normal speech development of a child and that the important skill that the two to four-year-old learns is rhythm, this seems the logical time for stuttering behavior to be learned. Some children begin to stutter after starting to school, but few begin at older ages.

5. A considerable number of individuals are reported to have stuttered during some period in their lives and to have "outgrown" the difficulty without

treatment. Many of these are reported by parents who say that "Johnny stuttered for a while when he was around three, but he outgrew it before he started to school." Usually, in such cases, Johnny will not remember this— unless he has been taught by his mother that he once stuttered. Another group of these former stutterers are those who were considered stutterers until old enough to remember all of the anxieties and negative responses that stutterers experience, and then in some way taught themselves to stop stuttering without the aid of any professional speech correctionist.

6. Practically all stutterers are originally diagnosed by laymen, not a speech clinician. Usually parents, again usually the mother, first consider the child to be stuttering, and it is not until after considerable concern and "help" that the child is brought to the speech clinician. This makes it very difficult for the researchers to describe the onset of stuttering.

7. Practically all children so diagnosed have spoken for from six months to several years without being regarded as defective in speech or as being abnormal. A few cases are reported to have "stuttered from the very beginning of speaking," but most parents can give some account of when the child "started to stutter." The remembered date is considerably after the date they give regarding "when he started to talk."

8. So-called stuttering children are not different from non-stuttering children with regard to birth injuries, diseases, intelligence, and general development. In general, they are normal children.

9. Stuttering children are like non-stuttering children with respect to handedness and handedness development. Contrary to earlier beliefs that stuttering resulted from change in handedness or that therapy involved determining handedness preference, there appears to be no evidence to support this opinion. Perhaps what is significant is that the rigid personality of a parent or teacher who would resort to such extremes as tying a child's left hand behind his back to force him to use his right hand is the kind of personality that could well cause sufficient anxiety and fear to promote non-fluent speech. These practices may well have given ample support for the belief that changing handedness would, indeed, cause stuttering.

10. Stuttering has been eliminated in a number of cases by means involving no recognized changes in the organic condition of the stutterer. In cases where therapy resulted in normal speech, physical examinations and monitoring of body functions revealed no organic changes.

11. Practically all stutterers experience fluency when they sing or speak in time to almost any form of rhythm or under conditions sufficiently noisy to mask their own voices; some act on stage without stuttering; most can talk to themselves, whisper, talk to pets, shout, speak with a dialect, and read in chorus fluently. In other words, there are conditions under which the stutterer is fluent. These may be divided into two groups of situations: (a)

conditions under which the stutterer hears himself abnormally as in choral reading, singing, or with interfering noise and (b) those in which he places no premium on fluency because he feels adequate as a speaker, as when talking to pets, small children, or himself.

12. More stuttering occurs on words that are nouns, verbs, adjectives, and adverbs; words that begin sentences; words that are longer than average; and words that begin with consonants. The word "the" would present less difficulty in the sentence, "I am going to the store" than the word would in "The store is nearby" and would present more difficulty in the last sentence than the word "a" in "A store is nearby." Words that are more important to the meaning of the sentence are more threatening. If the listener can guess the word from contextual cues, the stutterer is less apprehensive about conveying his message than if it cannot be guessed. For example, "I am reading a good bbbbbbb" may lead the listener to supply the intended "book" either understood or orally; but "My name is bbbbbbbb" can in no way assure the listener's being able to understand the intended message. The propositionality of the message is a significant factor.

13. Studies have found no differences between young adult stutterers and non-stutterers in ability to perform rapid, or rhythmical movement of lips, tongue, jaw, and breathing musculature. There has likewise been found no significant differences between the two groups with respect to heart rate, blood pressure, and basal metabolism.

14. More boys than girls stutter. Ratio reports vary from 10:1 to 2:1. The usually accepted ratio is 4:1. No conclusive explanation for this distribution difference with relation to sex has been found; yet there seems to be more than mere distribution significance with this respect. Males tend to experience a more severe form of stuttering than females, and females are more apt to "outgrow" their stuttering than males. Generally, in our culture males develop more slowly than females and are more susceptible to a considerable number of diseases and handicapping conditions, as well as to personal and social maladjustments. The factor of unequal competition may play a significant role in this unequal distribution factor, or there may be a genetic component, or both.

15. Stuttering behavior appears to run in families. Some have interpreted this to mean that stuttering is inherited genetically. It should be remembered, however, that a number of things tend to be inherited to which we attach no genetic significance. Being a Democrat, or being a Baptist tends to run in families; yet we don't say that these are genetically related. This is a social inheritance. Therefore, the fact that stuttering tends to run in families is not conclusive evidence that there is an organic basis for stuttering. Family discipline procedure, expectations, pressure, etc., often show similarities from generation to generation. If the conditions that caused a child to stutter in one generation are the kind of conditions that are present in subsequent genera-

tions, then the learning theory of stuttering origin is still not discounted by this familial tendency.

The Role of the Classroom Teacher

With the incidence of stuttering suggesting that fewer than one in every hundred school-age children stutters, it is to be expected that any teacher who teaches several years will encounter at least one stutterer. Usually, the stuttering child in the classroom is a real concern for the teacher, who is anxious not to make the child unduly self-conscious about his speech, not to have his peers make fun of him, not to make his speech worse, not to excuse poor academic work because of his speech handicap, etc. These are all negative goals, and, without positive goals, often his course of action is no action. Lacking information concerning what should be done, he does nothing. There are, however, both positive and negative suggestions for the teacher. Some of these are dependent on the stage of development that the stuttering behavior has reached. For this reason, some terms must be defined.

Terminology with reference to stuttering is difficult to describe because of differing opinions concerning the condition. Almost any list of terms would fit one explanation and fail to fit another. For the purpose of simplicity, terms will be kept to a minimum and confined to the most commonly encountered ones. The term "normal non-fluency" has already been used in describing the non-fluencies that we all experience, particularly those of the young child (not the beginning stutterer). The two terms, PRIMARY STUTTERER and SECONDARY STUTTERER are probably the most widely used to describe severity of stuttering behavior (3).

Primary stuttering refers to the easy, non-tense repetitions of the beginning stutterer. The speaker appears unaware of his disfluencies. Some authorities insist that this cannot be described as stuttering, since it is only when the speaker becomes aware of his disfluencies that he becomes a stutterer. Everyone who has observed stuttering in its various stages, however, realizes that there is a vast difference between the speech of the beginning stutterer and the confirmed one. So the term PRIMARY STUTTERER is used to describe the stutterer who has not acquired secondary characteristics associated with his stuttering, and it does not suggest an inevitable progression to a more severe stage of stuttering.

Secondary stuttering refers to the tense, non-fluent speech of the confirmed stutterer whose speech is associated with anxiety, fear, guilt, and perhaps hostility. Secondary stuttering is speech that is accompanied by secondary characteristics such as facial grimaces, tics, or other forms of spasmic movements either of the articulatory mechanism or of other parts of the body not ordinarily directly concerned with speech production. The stutterer has usually acquired these characteristics through years of practice and attempts to find speech aids, but the outcome has been negative, since the eye blinking, finger snapping, and the like are more distracting than his breaks in speech rhythm.

The term *transitional stage* (2) has been used to bridge the gap between the primary and secondary stages of stuttering development. This is the stage the stutterer goes through after he has become a stutterer but before he has acquired all of the secondary characteristics. He is aware of his stuttering and somewhat tense in many situations; he is beginning to fear certain words, speaking situations, or people. The careful observer, in considering how to handle the child, can draw his own conclusion relative to whether or not the child could be termed a secondary stutterer. If not, then we would use the suggestions for working with the primary stutterer.

Many lists have been compiled giving suggestions for both teachers and parents concerning how to work with stutterers. The author is aware of the dangers inherent in giving such lists, since stuttering is so variable and situational and since a reader may overgeneralize from lists of "Do's" and "Don'ts." Yet, there is merit in giving some concrete suggestions. In this book, an attempt has been made to divide the lists into suggestions for teachers of primary stutterers and those for teachers of secondary stutterers. Often there is no difference in recommended procedures. There is, however, one important difference. Where the primary stutterer is concerned, you would not want to call attention to his disfluency; but the secondary stutterer should learn to be able to talk about and not try to hide his stuttering. For a more detailed study of stuttering and what can be done, read *Stuttering: What It Is and What to Do about It* by Stanley Ainsworth in Cliffs Speech and Hearing Series.

Suggestions for Teachers of Primary Stutterers

THE GUIDING PRINCIPLE should be to understand the child's problem and accept him as a person of worth. More specifically, some DO's and DON'TS may help you to be aware of specifically helpful and harmful procedures. Many of these are simply good practices to use with all children, but, with the stutterer, they are urgent.

Do's for Teachers of Primary Stutterers

1. Become adjusted to the child's stuttering and react to it unemotionally and objectively. Imitation, impatience, embarrassment, or boredom on the part of the teacher causes the child to react unfavorably.

2. Create an atmosphere of ease and relaxation in the classroom. Rapid speech, loud commands, and military-like discipline may contribute to his disfluency.

3. See that you and those around the child are good listeners.

4. Allow the child to complete his sentences for himself. It is particularly disturbing for the stutterer to have words said for him or to be interrupted when he is trying to tell something.

5. Listen to the stutterer in a relaxed but interested manner. It is disturbing to him to have his listener look away while he is talking, to fidget and appear nervous, or to show relief when he gets out of a block, for example, to sigh as if relieved.

6. When the child is speaking, look at his eyes, not his lips.

7. Try to control the attitude of the class toward the stutterer and his speech. It may be necessary to instruct them privately not to stare or laugh. Explain that this is his present way of speaking, but that he should outgrow it and that they can help by listening quietly. Remember, too, that they are immature and that it is difficult for them to look entirely indifferent. The other children also need your patient understanding.

8. Increase the child's personality assets in every way. Neatness, cleanliness, and friendliness will do much to take attention away from his speech. Give him responsibilities that will build up self-esteem.

9. Assign him definite duties in the classroom that do not require speech responses. These must be REAL duties—not to be interpreted as "making a janitor" out of him.

10. Give him some leadership in recreational activities whenever possible.

11. Provide opportunities for choral reading. Stutterers usually experience fluency in this activity.

12. Give him opportunities to excel in those things that he does well. Help him overcome feelings of inferiority by literally bombarding him with feelings of confidence. Success is vital to a good self-concept, but it should be realistic. Give attention to positive characteristics and interests, but do not excuse poor work or conduct because of his stuttering. Instill in the child feelings of confidence and happiness in the classroom.

13. Some special consideration may be given the young stutterer during periods of oral recitation. If rapid oral drills are being used, the stutterer may be unobtrusively excluded.

14. Try to provide opportunities for speech with fluency. Observe the child and note times or situations in which he is more apt to be fluent. Give him as many ideal speech situations as possible.

15. Attempt to build up his self-confidence by the use of praise for work well done, especially art or written work. Praise should be genuine and should be merited—this does not refer to praise for being fluent.

16. Decrease the child's personality liabilities in every possible way. If he has any mannerisms or habits that are objectionable, they should be discussed unemotionally and objectively with him, and he should be helped to overcome them.

17. Phrase questions so that the stutterer can answer with short answers as opposed to long responses, which may result in tense blocks and undue attention from classmates. If he especially has trouble with oral questions, begin asking only questions that you are sure he knows the answer to and gradually increase the complexity of the child's spoken responses.

18. Control recitation activities so that expectancy fear does not build up prior to responding. Recitations that go from one child to another up one row of seats and down the next are somewhat threatening to all children, and particularly so to the stutterer, who can build up much anxiety waiting his turn. It would be better to skip around the room. Even such activities as calling the roll can create this anxiety for the child whose name begins with a letter near the end of the alphabetized roll. Skipping around in this activity is often helpful.

19. Provide special rhythmic exercises for the entire class such as marching, doing calisthenics to music, counting, clapping, and singing.

20. Let the stutterer use the hand of his choice.

21. Check the child's home life. Family bickering is upsetting to a child. By securing adequate knowledge of the background of the child's personality difficulties, the teacher may be able to help him to eliminate his worries and emotional problems.

22. After a particularly bad speech block, call the child's attention to something else, so that he will not fasten upon a specific sound as the cause of his speech difficulty and thereby establish a troublesome pattern of speech.

23. Give him a reasonable amount of attention and respect.

24. See that any health problems are given medical attention, not allowing the child to worry about his physical health nor to become overly obsessed with illness and faults.

25. Have a sincere and friendly interest in the child; give him affection.

Don'ts for Teachers of Primary Stutterers

1. Don't label a child a stutterer.

2. Don't make a great issue of speech. Treat it with lack of anxiety; listen in a calm relaxed manner; give the child time to say what he wishes to say without hurrying him.

3. Don't tell him to "stop and start over," to "take a deep breath," to "think before he speaks," to "take his time," or to swing his arms, swallow, or resort to any other such "helps."

4. Don't make fun of the stutterer nor show impatience, embarrassment, and boredom; don't criticize; don't accuse him of having a bad habit.
5. Don't have an atmosphere of tension in the classroom; avoid rapid speech and loud commands.
6. Avoid too severe discipline. Avoid ridicule or sarcasm as a disciplinary measure.
7. Don't expect too much of him.
8. Avoid discussing his shortcomings and weaknesses with others in his presence.
9. Put no pressures on speech. Don't criticize grammar, pronunciation, or posture when he is speaking.
10. Don't stress perfection in speech, but emphasize adjustment of the child to his environment regardless of speech defects.
11. Don't have him engage in activities that increase non-fluency, such as the use of flash cards and other speed drills. The emphasis on verbal competition increases the speech pressures. Use his written work as a measure of his knowledge. Substitute written recitations for oral responses if speaking causes embarrassment or aggravates his condition. Call for oral responses when you know that he knows the answers and will not be upset by the necessity to talk.
12. Don't assume that the stutterer is inferior mentally because he cannot express himself fluently. The average intelligence of stutterers has been found equal to that of the rest of the school population. Many times a stutterer says, "I don't know." only to avoid a speaking situation.
13. Don't call on the stutterer for oral work when it is evident that he is experiencing a particularly poor day. Stutterers have both good and bad speech days.
14. Don't display an attitude of pity or sympathy for the stutterer.
15. Don't praise the child for fluency. The normal speaker is not praised for fluent speech. The non-fluent child wants to be a normal person. Praise him for a correct answer or find some other REASON for praise.
16. Don't accept a wrong answer from him any more than you would from any other child. Sometimes we are guilty of not wanting to require further speech attempts and let a wrong answer go uncorrected rather than treating him normally with regard to academic work.
17. Don't change his handedness.
18. Don't let his speech difficulty become rewarding.

Obviously, there is much overlapping in the DO's and DON'TS, and many of them could be worded in either way. The point is that there are certain behaviors that the teacher can exhibit toward the stutterer that may either help him to be more fluent or increase his disfluency. The suggestions that are made for the classroom teacher of a secondary stutterer may be much the same as those for the primary stutterer in many respects. The basic difference is that while the primary stutterer may be only slightly aware of his disfluency or even unaware, the secondary stutterer is painfully aware of his speech problem. He has developed fear, avoidance, and anxiety associated with speaking situations.

Suggestions for Teachers of Secondary Stutterers

These suggestions apply to the individual who is known as a secondary stutterer, the one who is conscious of his non-fluency, who is developing secondary characteristics in his effort to make his speech more acceptable. This is the stutterer with whom you can and should discuss the problem of stuttering.

Some Do's

1. Avoid the terms "stuttering" and "stammering." Refer to the child's speech in terms of exactly what he does—hesitating, holding his breath, repeating sounds, prolonging sounds, eye blinking, etc.
2. Make no great issue of speech. Treat it as you would eyeglasses, dental braces, etc.
3. Accept his speech as *his* way of talking. The development of objectivity about stuttering is important. If he accepts his speech, he will not be nervous about it and will not fear speech situations.
4. Allow him to complete his sentence without being interrupted and without giving him the words.
5. Look at his eyes, not his lips.
6. Be a good listener. Have a sincere friendly interest in him. Consider his point of view. Win his confidence. Let him know that you are sincere in wanting to help him.
7. Talk to him about his problem. Find out his capabilities and his limitations: when he is fluent; when he is not.
8. Help him to develop a sense of humor about his speech, so that he can laugh at himself. If he is not sensitive, his classmates will not be as likely to tease him. They will be able to laugh with him rather than at him.
9. He should carry his fair share of conversation and classroom recitations, but some special consideration can be given him during periods of oral recitation. The stutterer may be unobtrusively excluded from some particularly tense or threatening recitations such as rapid oral drills, you also may be aware of particularly difficult days for him and avoid requir-

ing unnecessary oral recitation. On the other hand, stuttering should not serve the purpose of letting him get by or excusing him from work.

10. Control the attitude of the class. Instruct them privately not to stare, look bored, or laugh. Help them understand his speech problem and the important way in which they may aid his improvement. It may be helpful to solicit special assistance from a particular class leader.

11. Encourage him to excel in those studies in which he does well.

12. Have him read a passage aloud to you, in a slow, easy manner with light articulation. After he has read for the teacher, he may read to the class during one of the class reading sessions. It is characteristic of stutterers that with each succeeding reading of the same passage, they tend to become more fluent in that reading (adaptation).

13. Increase his personality assets. Give him responsibilities that will build up his self-esteem.

14. Encourage hobbies, extra reading, etc., that will make him a more interesting person, but encourage him not to hide or retreat into a hobby or reading to avoid contact with people.

15. Encourage his classmates to befriend him and not make fun of him. Discourage jokes, songs, or stunts that make fun of stutterers.

16. Encourage him to talk. Fearing speaking, he probably has a tendency to avoid speech situations. Encouraging him to speak often will help him overcome that fear, but never force him to speak.

17. Assign roles in dramatizations in which he uses pronounced differences in speech patterns, for example, an assumed accent. Most stutterers can do this type of speech activity with little difficulty.

18. Teachers in a school system should confer with each other, the principal, and parents about how to proceed with each case, so that all who come in contact with him will be supportive of the manner in which he is being treated.

19. Remember that he is a person.

In conclusion, if there is a speech clinician in the school system, refer the stutterer for therapy. Confer with the clinician for information concerning how you can help and also in order to give the clinician insight relative to the child's classwork and peer relations. Get to know his family so that you may make recommendations to them. If there is no speech clinician, you cannot be expected to have either the time or the training to provide therapy for the difficult problem of stuttering, but you can do many of the things that will help him feel better about himself and, hopefully, to become a better speaker.

Chapter 6

Voice Disorders

Voice disorders occur far less frequently than do problems of articulation, but those that do occur in the school-age population tend to be ignored unless they are very dramatic. Some speech clinicians tend to shy away from voice problems because of their feelings of inadequacy in altering a person's voice. Most classroom teachers do not recognize vocal disturbances and they may likewise be overlooked by some speech clinicians. Fox says that "of all the skills a speech clinician now has available for the management of vocal problems, perhaps the most valuable asset is awareness . . . without that particular skill many voice problems go unrecognized, unidentified, and untreated" (52).

The problem of correcting vocal disorders is further complicated by the resistance of people to voice therapy or to the idea of changing their voices. Your voice is probably the most personal thing about you, and although you may be interested in self-improvement it may be a bit too threatening to your ego to have someone attempt to change your voice; hence resistance to therapy.

Voice therapy is a very specialized skill and should not be attempted by a non-professional speech clinician. Mild, bad habit type vocal inefficiencies may be dealt with in the classroom, however, and all children as well as the teacher will benefit from attention given to more efficient use of voice.

Disorders

Voice disorders have to do with faults in *pitch*, *quality*, *loudness*, and *time*. The cause may be physical, learned, or psychological. Whatever the voice problem noted, the individual must have an examination by a laryngologist prior to voice therapy. The possibility of a pathology of the vocal folds must be explored. With a clearance from the laryngologist, the speech clinician will initiate therapy designed to eliminate the problem or to teach compensatory voice use.

Pitch

Pitch should be appropriate for the age, sex, and size of the speaker. Our unconscious awareness of this may be evident in our shock or surprise when we hear a very high-pitched voice come from a large man, a masculine sounding voice come from a small woman, or an adult sounding voice come from a small child. Such speakers are often embarrassed and self-conscious about their voices; they may suffer social penalties having far-reaching social, economic, educational, and vocational consequences; yet they may go through life without help. Two important factors contribute to the latter. First, many people are unaware that such therapy is available or appropriate. Second, the feeling that one's voice is one's personality causes people to resist therapy aimed at voice change.

One female university student with a high-pitched, thin voice who was usually mistaken on the telephone for a preschooler came to the speech clinic for therapy. Progress was slow, however, because of her fear that changing her voice would change her personality. Another case with the opposite problem of a low-pitched voice requested therapy because she was consistently mistaken for a man when talking over the telephone; yet she did not want to change her voice in ordinary face-to-face conversation because of what her friends might think or say.

In a discussion of pitch, two terms that must be understood are *optimum pitch* and *habitual pitch*. Everyone has a pitch that is best for him. This is called *optimum pitch*, and it is the pitch at which an individual's voice functions most efficiently. This does not mean a fixed pitch, but rather the median or average pitch at which the vocal mechanism functions best. *Habitual pitch* refers to the pitch we usually use—again, not a fixed pitch, but the pitch at which we ordinarily initiate phonation or the median around which our pitch variations tend to cluster. Optimum and habitual pitch should be about the same. If there is much difference between the two, then the speaker is using an inappropriate pitch that may be both unpleasant to listen to and also harmful to the speaker's vocal health.

The physical determinants of pitch are the size, shape, and material of the sound-producing mechanism. In a stringed musical instrument this may be the length, thickness, and elasticity of the string. The same principle applies to the vocal folds. The longer, thicker folds of the male produce lower-pitched sounds than the shorter, thinner folds of the female. The age, health, and makeup of the folds will affect their elasticity, thus altering pitch.

The mechanism itself is not the sole determinant of pitch. We can adjust the pitch by altering the amount of tension. With the stringed musical instrument, we do this by tightening the string, thus increasing the tension. With our voices, we increase the tension by stretching or elongating the vocal folds. Ordinarily these adjustments are made to give variety. If, however, we habitually use a pitch that is significantly above or below our optimum pitch, we have a voice disorder involving an inappropriate pitch. A speech clinician can ascertain the optimum pitch during a voice evaluation. A classroom teacher should probably rely on her educated judgment concerning the acceptability of most children's pitch. For the child with an unusual pitch, the teacher should consult a professional speech clinician for evaluation. A word of caution is in order here. The classroom teacher should encourage pleasing voices; however, the correction of a voice problem should be handled with care. A pitch change resulting in an effortful, breathy voice may be harmful.

Quality

Voice quality is that which gives each voice individuality. How do you recognize a person just from a simple "Hello" on the telephone? Voices are so distinctive that they can be distinguished by voiceprints just as people can be identified from fingerprints. Basically, however, there are qualities that can be described as *harsh, hoarse, strident, metallic, aspirate, breathy, nasal, denasal,* and *normal.* Terms describing quality are often difficult to define, since a voice that sounds hoarse to one listener may be described by another listener as guttural, throaty, or pleasing.

Some deviant voice qualities are extremely noticeable and easily recognized. A voice that is hypernasal readily calls attention to itself whether the nasality is organically caused, as in the case of the cleft palate speaker, or if it is a functional problem, as in the case of certain regional speech that has a distinct nasal quality. The same is true of hyponasality (denasality), which may result from such conditions as nasal congestion or enlarged adenoidal tissue that closes off the nasal cavity, preventing the nasal resonance necessary for the *m, n,* and *ng* phonemes.

Intensity

The intensity or loudness of voice is self-evident. Most people at some time have experienced a temporary loss of voice caused by excessive yelling or too loud talking. You may have lost your voice in connection with an upper respiratory infection causing laryngitis. Permanent aphonia (no voice) may result from growths on the vocal folds that prevent their approximation, from paralysis, or, in cases of surgical removal of the larynx, there would be no normal voice-producing apparatus.

Not all problems of intensity are of organic nature. A normal vocal mechanism can produce a voice that would be considered ordinarily too loud and also one that would be considered too weak for normal speech. The loudness of our voices should be controlled by the speaking situation. Usually, speakers do this quite unconsciously. When we yell at players on the football field, we do so with great intensity; when we call on a bereaved family at a funeral home, we usually speak in a very quiet voice. Sometimes, children do not learn this kind of monitoring without some special help. You may have known a child who always spoke so softly that he could scarcely be heard or one who always talked as if he were attempting to be heard above the roar of a crowded subway. If the problem is not organic, the speech clinician may enlist the aid of the classroom teacher in helping a particular child become aware of the loudness yardstick by which we usually gauge our voice intensity and in helping him to learn to monitor his own loudness. Problems with an organic origin, such as those associated with a hearing disability, must be dealt with in terms of the specific disability.

Time

Time has to do with the rate of our speech, or the tempo of our speech. Rate is influenced by emotions, situational factors, basic drives, intelligibility, personality, breathing, and phrasing (52). Disturbed rate can be organically caused, as in the case of cerebral palsy or Parkinson's disease. Rate can vary dramatically and remain effective. It is only when rate interferes with the efficiency of our speech for communication that it is of concern. The problem of an excessively slow rate is seldom encountered in the school-age population, but many children speak too rapidly. Classroom instruction can be interesting for children and beneficial in helping them learn to use an appropriate rate. This may involve such activities as role playing or choral reading.

Causes

As already suggested, voice disorders may be considered to be either organic or functional. Although we use these terms, it is difficult to dichotomize causes in this way. For instance, a cleft palate speaker's defective voice is considered to be of organic origin, and it certainly is. Yet this individual may speak with a quieter voice than he may otherwise use because of his self-consciousness about his nasal voice. The result may be a voice that is insufficient in intensity and perhaps also too high pitched (both functional problems for him) in addition to the organically caused nasality. Furthermore, a functionally caused problem, such as a voice that is loud and harsh associated with an aggressive personality, may result in physical changes in the vocal folds, causing an organic voice disorder. With these considerations in mind, the following brief description will help point out the multiplicity of causes.

Functional Causes

Psychological factors may cause a voice problem, ranging from the very severe problem of hysterical aphonia (psychologically unable to produce voice) to the thin, whiny voice of a shy child. The severe problems are for the psychiatrist and the speech pathologist. The milder problems may also require voice therapy, but sometimes they may be dealt with, at least in part, in the classroom. Often the reason for the voice disturbance no longer exists, but the bad habit persists. For instance, the child who developed a whining or complaining sounding voice during a long period of illness may now be physically fit yet continue to use the unpleasant voice.

Unsuitable pitch levels may be caused by imitation, timidity, or habit persisting from a time when the vocal habit was acquired. An inappropriate pitch is often interpreted by the listener to be some other problem. For instance, a voice described as being a thin voice may actually be too high pitched, giving it the thin-sounding quality. Since pitch is determined by the tension and mass of the vibrator, the person who constantly speaks in an excessively high pitch is constantly keeping his vocal folds tensed and stretched. The person, however, who speaks in a low-pitched monotone is constantly keeping his folds pushed down into an abnormally short length. Make a sound such as *ah* as low pitched as you can. Now make a sound such as *ee* as high pitched as you can. Note the difference in the muscle tension in your neck as well as vocal postures. Imagine always talking at either end of your pitch range! How tiring to you; how tiresome to the listener.

A large proportion of all voice problems are associated with vocal hyperfunction or vocal abuse. The previous example of laryngitis that may be caused by excessive or loud talking or yelling is a well-known example. Laymen, however, often consider any indication of a growth on the vocal folds as being purely organic in origin. True, some of them are, but there are swellings or formations that are caused by vocal abuse. These are usually vocal *nodules* which may be called singer's nodes, preacher's nodes, teacher's nodes, etc., depending on who has them. Nodules may occur on either or both vocal folds at the point where the folds slam together with the greatest force. They usually start somewhat like a bruise and can be reversed with vocal rest or voice therapy while they are in the formative stage. If not corrected early, they continue to become more callous-like until they are too hard to respond to voice therapy. Surgical removal is the procedure for nodules of long duration. This may be followed by voice therapy to teach the individual a less abusive use of his voice, which in turn should prevent their recurrence. *Hematomas* are much the same as nodules except that they hemorrhage rather than become callous in nature. Treatment follows the same pattern as for nodules.

Contact ulcers constitute another type of physical problem with a functional cause. These occur primarily when the speaker is using an excessively low-pitched voice. As would be expected, they are more common in males than in females. The ulcers form on the edge of the posterior portion of the vocal folds, become crater-like, and form granulated layers, producing a protrusion from the fold. This protrusion prevents proper closure, with a resultant hoarseness.

Breathing may be associated with inefficient time. Although there may be differences in the place of maximum movement during breathing, generally this does not impair voice production. Some people may exhibit this maximum movement in the abdominal region indicating very deep breathing, while others vary from lower to upper thoracic breathing. Any of these is adequate for normal voice. If, however, the speaker uses clavicular breathing, he is not making efficient use of his breath for speech purposes and the result may be some disturbance in time. Clavicular breathing can be identified by observing the speaker. If he raises his shoulders to inhale, he probably has very shallow clavicular breathing.

Another problem associated with time includes the person who takes a breath and speaks until he seems to run out of air, then inhales again regardless of the meaningfulness of the place of pause. He has not learned to program his inhalations with regard to enhancing the meaning of what he is saying. Sometimes a person's speech is disturbed by audible inhalation or by exhaling much of his air supply and then attempting to speak on the residual air.

Organic Causes

Teachers in junior high and secondary schools will encounter varying degrees of adolescent voice change, which is a secondary sex characteristic. The voice change may be accompanied by some degree of apprehension on the part of the young man. Actually, what happens is a matter of growth. Male and female larynges are not too different in size until the adolescent growth spurt of the male larynx. During a short period of time, the male larynx increases one-third in size. The speaker, having learned how to phonate to achieve the intended sound, suddenly finds that an unexpected sound emerges when he initiates phonation. His attempts to "correct" result in over-correction or adjustment, giving a sliding effect or a break. Some speakers adjust quickly and effortlessly to their new-sized larynx; others find the adjustment more difficult. Both boys and girls experience some lowering of pitch during adolescence, but girls' voices lower only a few notes, while boys' voices lower about an octave.

Other disorders of organic origin include laryngitis caused by disease. A common offender is chronic upper respiratory infection, with its associated chronic postnasal drip. Paralysis, too, may involve either or both vocal folds, resulting in voice disorders varying from hoarseness to complete aphonia.

Growths occurring on the vocal folds in the form of tumors may be either benign or malignant. *Polyps* are the most common kind of benign tumor. Others include *fibromas*, *papillomas*, and *cysts*. These are not caused by vocal abuse and treatment consists of surgical removal. The only means of distinguishing benign tumors from malignant ones is by laboratory analysis. Malignant tumors are rare in children, but they do occur. They occur most frequently among older males. If detected early, surgical removal may not involve complete amputation of the larynx resulting in no means of making normal voice. Hoarseness is usually an early symptom and should receive the attention of a laryngologist, since prognosis is excellent in the early stages. If complete removal of the malignancy requires excision of the entire larynx, the patient must breathe through an opening made in his neck (stoma). With no means of getting pulmonary air from his lungs into his mouth, he must learn a means of alaryngeal speech.

Excision of the larynx, although rare, may be necessitated by causes other than cancer. An accident may result in such a necessity. Endocrine disorders constitute yet another organic cause of voice disorders. Diseases such as emphysema cause a loss of respiratory efficiency, which may force the speaker to speak in short phrases, resulting in a disorder of time.

Therapy

Although the treatment of voice disorders is a highly specialized skill and may take different procedural steps, it can be said that a large majority of these problems are corrected with procedures aimed at reducing hyperfunction of the vocal mechanism. Probably the first step will be to convince the person that he has a problem. The individual who went to a laryngologist because of persistent hoarseness and was told that he had created nodules on his vocal folds through abuse may be motivated to alter his voice. Simply learning what the problem is and that it may be eliminated through vocal retraining, that in turn should prevent its recurrence, is sufficient motivation for many people. On the other hand, the person who has someone recommend that he seek therapy because his voice is unpleasant or has a distracting quality often is not so motivated. It is not that he does not want to have a pleasant voice, rather that he doesn't really believe that his voice is unpleasant to all people. At any rate, there is little that the clinician can do for the person who is not convinced that he has a problem.

General remedial procedures will include setting a goal to be achieved, exercises designed to eliminate the specific problem, and help with self-monitoring. The goal is to have the speaker transfer the desired manner of voice production to ordinary conversational speech. Often this phase is complicated by so-called friends of the voice case who tell the speaker that his new voice doesn't sound like him, that they liked the way he talked before, or that his old voice was his personality. Family and friends may reject the new voice. See *Clinical Management of Voice Disorders* by Donna Fox in Cliffs Speech and Hearing Series for specific therapy techniques.

The Role of the Classroom Teacher

As previously stated, the classroom teacher will not attempt to provide voice therapy for a pathological voice problem, but he should be aware of the implications of deviant vocal production. A child who is persistently hoarse should be referred to a physician, preferably a laryngologist. A child with either nasal or denasal speech should also be seen by a medical doctor. Therefore, one of the classroom teacher's major contributions to voice improvement may be in his becoming "tuned in" to voice quality and learning to recognize deviant voices. He must also be prepared to work with the child's parents to inform them of the child's need to modify his voice.

The classroom teacher can also do other things. To aid the speech clinician, he can help to arouse the child's motivation to improve his vocal function. Class activities to create an awareness of the part that our voices play in interpersonal relations and ways of effecting changes may become a part of the language program. Games that allow children to try to identify classmates will help children become aware of the distinctive features of voices. Probably the most effective tool at the disposal of the classroom teacher is the tape recorder.

The teacher may be able to improve the everyday speaking of the child. If the child exhibits hoarseness from vocal abuse, the speech clinician may ask the teacher's assistance in helping the child learn to monitor and chart the times when he does this. If the child has a functionally breathy voice, the clinician may enlist the aid of the teacher in putting the child in selected situations where he must speak louder in order to be heard. Sometimes the help is in the form of counteracting shyness and timidity and encouraging confidence and poise. It may involve helping children understand the importance of variety and rate in making their speech interesting as well as understandable. Specific suggestions for emphasizing voice in the speech-improvement program include:

1. *Help the child hear himself.*

The tape recorder is the best tool for this, but be sure that it is of good quality so that children are able to recognize each others' voices. Also, using devices such as clapping their hands over their ears or putting a paper bag over their heads while talking may help them hear themselves. Have them experiment with various pitch and loudness levels while listening to themselves in this way.

2. *Compare voices.*
Play guessing games where children must identify each other from only a word or two. Have two speakers say the same word and decide which is higher pitched or which is louder.

3. *Identify pleasing voices.*
Give examples of different voices and ask children to identify them as "a pretty voice" or "one that is not pretty." Use examples of a whiny voice, a gravelly voice, a nasal voice, a pleasant voice.

4. *Note pitch change.*
Role-play the story of "The Three Bears" and talk about the voices of Father Bear, Mother Bear, and Baby Bear. Use a vowel slide drawn on the chalkboard, by drawing a playground type slide on the board with a vowel at the top. As you move a pointer up or down the slide, have the children produce the vowel and raise or lower the pitch according to the movement of the pointer and to the speed of the movement.

5. *Teach tone changes.*
Read a few lines from a poem such as "The Raven" in the slow, mournful voice that is usually used, then read a few lines from "To a Meadow Lark" in the usual lilting voice. Reverse the procedure and ask the children if "The Raven" sounds as well read in a lilting voice or "To a Meadow Lark" in a mournful voice. Let children read a sentence to express meaning, for example, "Come to mommie," "Naughty boy," "Run for your life," "Let me tell you a secret," etc. Discuss the effect of voice on meaning.

6. *Teach use of volume.*
Whisper. Speak from a stage of a large auditorium. Role-play stories such as "The Three Billy Goats Gruff."

7. *Teach breath control.*
Phonate an *s* sound for one second, for two seconds, for three seconds, for four seconds. Count to 20 on one breath. Read a paragraph and mark where you inhaled.

8. *Practice in use of force.*
Tell the child that there is something on his hand and to use just enough force to blow it off—a feather, a piece of paper, a piece of cardboard, a piece of chalk. Use the "be quiet" sound to tell the entire class to be quiet.

9. *Teach resonance.*

Pretend you have a cold. Occlude the nares to make yourself sound denasal. Have children read a phrase such as "how now brown cow" and pretend to swallow a hard-boiled egg with each vowel. Have them read the same phrase with a very small mouth opening. Feel the vibration on the nose while humming; while saying *ah*.

Suggestions for Helping Children Keep a Healthy Voice

1. It is generally agreed that misuse of the voice is the most common cause of voice problems in children. This misuse can take many forms such as:
   a. Yelling and excessively loud talking. This does not affect all children in the same way, but if a child has hoarseness, then such abuse should be discouraged.
   b. Such unnatural uses of the voice as imitating cars, motor boats, machine guns, and the like may contribute to voice problems because of the unusual strain on the voice.
   c. Cheerleading, singing, and acting may add to the problem and should be carefully supervised.
   d. When a child has a sore throat and hoarseness, reduce all vocal activities, including talking, to a bare minimum. In the case of severe laryngitis, vocal activity should be discontinued until the voice is healthy.
   e. Special consideration should be given the boy undergoing adolescent voice change. Be patient and sympathetic; do not put him in embarrassing situations; perhaps discourage singing during this time; and above all do not encourage him to maintain his little boy voice. If he has particular difficulty you may want to discuss with him the physical aspect of what is happening or you may want to get help from a speech pathologist.
2. Good physical health is important to a sound, healthy voice. Voice problems may be caused by such conditions as:
   a. Upper respiratory infections that may result in swollen, inflamed membranes. Repeated colds should receive medical attention.
   b. Coughing is especially abusing to vocal folds. Repeated or prolonged coughs should receive attention.
   c. Allergies tend to weaken the tissues of the larynx and make them more susceptible to damage from use or misuse of the voice.
   d. Infected tonsils may spread infection to the laryngeal area.
   e. General poor health tends to be reflected in one's voice. We are familiar with the observation of "You don't sound as if you feel well."

3. Emotional problems also show up in one's voice. A normally speaking child may develop hoarseness under conditions of unusual strain. Sometimes these factors involve:
   a. Sibling rivalry in which one child may be trying to keep up with, compete with, or take attention away from a brother or sister who may be older, more aggressive, more talented, or for some reason poses a threat to the child may result in undue tension in speaking situations. Parental favoritism may contribute to this.
   b. Disrupted home and family relationships may contribute to emotional problems that may emerge as voice problems.
4. Individual differences make it difficult to understand why one child may engage in a given behavior with no apparent adverse effects on his voice while another child suffers a severe penalty for shouting, coughing, or excessive talking. Being aware of the causes of voice problems, tuned in to them, and aware of remedial procedures should do much to help all children learn to use their voices most efficiently.

Chapter 7

Special Problems

Although the speech characteristics associated with disabilities such as cleft palate, cerebral palsy, and aphasia may involve any of the previously discussed disorders of language, articulation, voice, and rhythm, these organic disorders occur with sufficient frequency and severity to merit special consideration. Speech therapy needed by these individuals will differ in some ways from therapy given for faulty articulation and voice. The basic problem presents unique involvements.

Cleft Palate

A facial cleft is an abnormality involving an opening, or cleft, in the structures of the oral cavity, lips, or nasal cavity. Ordinarily this is a developmental failure (prebirth) but an accident at birth or following birth can cause a cleft, or abnormal opening. Although incidence figures vary from one study to another, most indicate that about one baby out of every 750 live births is born with a facial cleft. This means that he is born with an opening in the roof of his mouth (cleft palate) or in his lip (cleft lip) or both. The term *cleft palate* is often used in the broad sense to include both conditions.

The birth of a cleft palate offspring is a particularly traumatic experience for the parents because of the child's appearance. After the initial shock, however, parents usually adjust rather quickly for, unlike conditions such as cerebral palsy and mental retardation, facial clefts are correctable with surgical and therapeutic management.

In order to understand the possibility of this developmental failure, it is helpful to know something of the development of the embryo. During the early weeks of fetal development, the various parts of the body begin to take on the appearance that they will have at birth. The first evidence of the upper lip and the hard and soft palate appear about the sixth week of fetal development. Over a period of several weeks the upper lip and upper jaw are formed by structures growing in from each side and meeting at the midline, with a third portion growing downward from the nasal region. The roof of the mouth is formed in much the same way, with the bony hard palate in the

103

anterior (front) part of the mouth and the soft palate posterior to it. The fusion of all these structures starts with the lip and proceeds posteriorly, ending with the soft palate. By the end of the twelfth week this fusion is complete, and the nasal cavity is separated from the oral cavity by the completely formed hard and soft palates. If there is a disturbance in fetal development during this period when the face is developing, the result is some sort of incomplete fusion, or cleft.

Obviously, the time and extent of the disturbance affect the kind and amount of the cleft. If a disturbance occurs early and lasts throughout the period when the fusion is taking place, the child will be born with a cleft of both lip and palate, perhaps on both sides. A disturbance occurring early in the fusion period and not lasting long may result in a child with a cleft of the lip but with a normal palate. A disturbance occurring later in the fusion period will affect the palate.

Causes

Although specific causes for each cleft are often impossible to determine, certain causal factors are known. Cleft lip is more dependent on heredity than is cleft palate. Many observations of causes have been made on lower animals and may not give adequate explanations of human malformations, but they suggest that similar factors may cause facial anomalies in human infants. Certain vitamin deficiencies in pregnant rats have been shown to produce cleft palate offspring. Radiation, infectious diseases, and certain drugs have produced the same effect in laboratory studies.

Special Needs

The most immediate need for the newborn cleft palate baby is feeding, which presents a particular problem because of his inability to nurse normally. Cleft palate babies seem more susceptible to colds than other children, and they tend to have a higher than normal incidence of ear infections and defective hearing. The health of the baby and the closure of the cleft usually get major early attention. Concern for his speech may be delayed until other problems have been solved. In some cases, this postponement has meant failure to give adequate attention to speech needs during crucial speech-development years.

The rehabilitation of the cleft palate child is complicated and involves many specialists. For this reason, a cleft palate team works together from the time of the child's birth to plan and coordinate the child's habilitation. The team consists of the pediatrician, plastic surgeon, orthodontist, speech pathologist, social worker, audiologist, otolaryngologist, psychologist, prosthodontist, and perhaps others. The goal of therapy is to make the cleft palate child as normal speaking, normal looking, and normal functioning as possible.

The majority of the cleft palate cases have completed the necessary surgery and have had some type of speech correction before they enter the first grade. In addition, they may have been fitted with a prosthetic appliance to aid in palatal function, and many of them are receiving extensive dental care. Such is not always the case. Some individuals go through life with an unrepaired cleft. The tragedy of this is there is no need for any child, no matter how indigent the family nor how remote their residence to be denied the rehabilitation services of the cleft palate team. Although the total rehabilitation is expensive, the service is available through the crippled children's division of the state health departments. Even so, not all cleft palate children receive the available help. Sometimes ignorance, superstition, and other "reasons" not only prevent the family from seeking help but may actually cause them to resist that which is offered.

The Role of the Classroom Teacher

If a classroom teacher encounters a child whose speech is suggestive of a cleft palate, he should not merely assume that the child's speech is as adequate as possible. The child should be referred to the school speech clinician for an evaluation and/or therapy. If the school does not have a speech clinician, an examination by a doctor or other specialist would help determine the cause of the child's defective speech. In addition, the child's school records may be helpful in understanding his problem.

If it is found that a child has an unrepaired cleft, perhaps the most important contribution that the teacher could make would be to help the parents see and understand how and why their child needs help and to assist them in following through with contacts and appointments. The child will probably have articulatory errors because of his inability to effect the necessary closure between the oral and nasal cavities for normal articulation. He will, likewise, probably have a nasal quality to his voice and may have nasal emission (air coming out his nose audibly). If the cleft has been closed, however, then the teacher's role will be that of aiding the child in his psychological adjustment, as well as fostering good speech, voice, and language development.

Speech therapy for the cleft palate child is challenging for the trained speech pathologist; therefore, the classroom teacher will not be expected to provide therapy, but he can learn more about the problem, work with parents, and carry out any suggestions that a professional speech clinician may give him for aiding the child with his speech. For information the teacher could contact the crippled children's division of the state health department, a nearby university speech clinic, the American Cleft Palate Association, or the American Speech and Hearing Association.

If there is a school speech clinician, the classroom teacher can be a great help in providing information about the child's speech in his daily classes, his reaction when people have difficulty understanding him, his relations with his peers, and his academic program. The teacher may be asked to carry out some direct work on the child's speech or to reinforce and supplement other phases of the remedial program. The precise things that the classroom teacher can best do will vary from one child to another. Teacher and therapist are limited only by their imagination and resources.

When considering the cleft palate child, it is important to keep in mind that we are not talking about an abnormal child but rather a normal child with a special problem. There are four factors that are important in rehabilitation: (a) the age of the child, (2) cooperation of the parents, (3) adequacy of repair or prosthetic device, and (4) the child and his cleft. First, the speech therapist needs to be involved with the child's speech and language development as early as possible. The first phase of therapy should be parent training, to instruct them in the ways to stimulate speech and language. Second, parent cooperation is essential. It has been said that cleft palate children develop into patient children because of the many hours they must sit with an open mouth allowing the different specialists to observe their deformity. Their parents deserve some credit for being patient people also. It takes much time, patience, and devotion to the task of habilitation in order for parents to keep the many appointments, carry out the many special tasks, and give their child the special help that he needs.

Adequacy of repair or prosthetic device is also a significant factor. If the prosthesis doesn't fit, if the repair doesn't create an adequate palate, if there is a breakdown of structures, no speech pathologist can expect success. Finally, abilities and problems the child presents to the therapist or teacher are important. The extent of the cleft, the child's intelligence, his motivation to improve, and his mental health all have an impact on the success of habilitation procedures.

Many improvements have been made in the last few decades that have bettered the life of the cleft palate child. Surgical correction has been improved, prosthodontic and orthodontic procedures have been improved, and improved techniques have been developed by the speech pathologists, but the child must acquire a positive attitude before any of the specialists' help can be optimally effective. This positive attitude, so vital in the child's life, can be acquired by the child only through his parents' attitude and willingness to help, and through the teacher's ability to acquire and maintain an attitude of friendliness in the classroom. It is most important that the cleft palate child be accepted by society the first time that he is introduced to society and that society is introduced to him. For many, this introduction occurs in the school setting.

For a more complete study of the cleft palate child and his speech, read *Cleft Palate and Associated Speech Characteristics* by Raymond Massengill, Jr., and Phyllis P. Phillips, in Cliffs Speech and Hearing Series.

Cerebral Palsy

Congenital cerebral palsy refers to a condition caused by injury to the motor area of the brain before, during, or immediately after birth. Again, the severely involved child is not likely to be found in the regular classroom. Cerebral palsied children may have one or a number of associated conditions such as a visual problem, hearing disorder, and mental retardation, but it is the impairment of the neuromuscular control that distinguishes the child with cerebral palsy from other groups of handicapped children.

Types

Cerebral palsy is not a disease; it is not a unitary condition resulting from a single set of circumstances; instead, it is a group of conditions. The most common type of cerebral palsy is the *spastic* type, which makes up about 65 percent of the total. In general, the motor activity of these children is characterized by jerky, labored, and uneven movement when trying to carry out any voluntary act. The next most common type is the *athetoid* type, which makes up about 20 percent of the total. These children exhibit involuntary slow, writhing movements that increase when they try to carry out any voluntary act. The third group, the *ataxic*, makes up only about 5 percent of the total. The chief symptom is lack of coordination and balance. The remaining 5 percent is made up of other types such as *atonic*, *tremor*, and *rigidity*. There may also be *mixed* types.

Causes

Causes of cerebral palsy are many, but they may be classified as *prenatal*, *perinatal*, or *postnatal*. The brain may fail to develop properly during embryonic life. Such prenatal causes include illnesses of the mother such as rubella (German measles) during the early months of pregnancy, maternal bleeding, and metabolic disturbances. Perinatal conditions are those occurring at birth, such as cerebral hemorrhage, and cerebral anoxia. The most common postnatal causes are injury, infections, illness, and poisons. Any condition that cuts off or sharply reduces the oxygen supply to the child's brain and occurs shortly before, during, or after birth may cause cerebral palsy.

Incidence figures on cerebral palsy vary considerably, but perhaps there are about three or four cases out of every 1,000 population with one out of every 200 live births being cerebral palsied. This figure has risen in the last half of this century. A possible explanation for this rise is that a number of babies who are now surviving the condition that made them cerebral palsied would have died, had they been born during the first half of the century. Hopefully, the incidence of cerebral palsy will be reduced with improved immunization against measles and rubella, as well as with new knowledge that will come about through future research.

The Role of the Classroom Teacher

Perhaps one of the problems of the cerebral palsied child with which the teacher may be most helpful is that of attitudes. Because of the motor involvement and the associated staggering gait and slurred, labored speech, cerebral palsied people are often misunderstood and likewise mistreated. They may be considered mentally retarded, drunk, on drugs, or as having some kind of seizure. Therefore, helping the cerebral palsied child adjust to the group may be an important role for the teacher. It may be necessary to talk with the other members of the class at a time when he is not in the room in order to help them understand and accept his problem. Often there is no need for this, but the sensitive and observant teacher will know if it is needed. It is well to enlist the aid of classmates, since they may need to give assistance with some of the regular activities. Understanding, not sympathy, is needed, and the teacher is probably the one who will set the tone for the entire class.

Almost anything that can be said along this line may sound like an outworn cliché; yet the meaning of the words is very important. Many people concentrate on the differences—the physical impairment—so much that they seem unable to get beyond them. The handicapped child is especially in need of being accepted as a person, of people getting to know him rather than his handicap, of knowing warm friendships rather than pity.

It should be understood that there may be associated problems, since the injuries to the brain that caused the motor impairment rarely affect only the control of muscles. Important sensory and perceptual disturbances may also be present. The exact incidence of mentally retarded cerebral palsied individuals is difficult to determine, since the sensory, perceptual, motor, and speech difficulties of these children make intelligence testing very difficult. Perhaps as many as 50 percent are mentally deficient. There is also a high incidence of hearing and vision problems. Perhaps one-fourth of them have impaired hearing and more than one-half have visual problems (13).

It is incorrect to talk about cerebral palsied speech, since a cerebral palsied person can have adequate speech and since their speech varies according to the type and extent of the condition. It is true, however, that the large majority of them do have defective speech. The speech disorder is often more than just the inability to achieve normal articulation and normal resonance. They frequently have an overall language problem involving difficulty in learning to comprehend, to talk, to read, and to write. It is difficult to separate the learning disabilities from the environmentally induced problems. Families often overindulge or overprotect as well as unconsciously reject the cerebral palsied child.

These children, like those with cleft palate, are under the habilitative direction of a team. The cerebral palsy team is made up of the physician, the physical therapist, the occupational therapist, the psychologist, the social worker, and the speech clinician. Again, the classroom teacher would not be expected to have the training, the time nor professional responsibility to undertake speech remediation with this child, but, depending on the child's involvement, the teacher may be able to provide him with some speech stimulation or to carry out the instructions of a speech clinician.

There are two other things that the classroom teacher should keep in mind. The cerebral palsied child often needs some special consideration. Although you want him to participate in all regular classroom activities, you must remember that he has difficulty with all motor-involved activities. This is the nature of his disability; therefore, one positive consideration may be to make things a little easier for him. This is not to say that he is excused from duties, but rather that such minor arrangements as seating may make a difference in his day. For instance, simply assigning him a seat near the pencil sharpener or where he does not have to walk as far when going to lunch may appear to be small considerations, indeed, but they may mean a great deal in the total activity of the day.

A second point to remember is that relaxation is one of the child's main difficulties. At least some of his muscles are nearly always unnaturally tense. He will be helped if the classroom routine can be arranged so that he is provided with frequent opportunities to relax. In some cases, a special seat may be provided to help him be more comfortable and relaxed in the classroom. He may need some special equipment. For instance, a child who cannot hold a pencil may be able to use an electric typewriter. Remember, too, that cerebral palsied children speak better when relaxed; therefore, the more comfortable the classroom atmosphere, the more efficient will be speech.

Special considerations should be given to the adolescent cerebral palsied student. In many instances, they may make satisfactory adjustments until they reach this age and then develop severe emotional problems. Many normal adolescents have problems in adjustment during the adolescent period, and for the child with multiple handicaps in locomotion, speech, and other areas, the problem of developing satisfactory relationships with the opposite sex may overshadow his other handicaps. School dances, first dates, sports, learning to drive a car, and acceptable speech are examples of the ways that he is left out of the "important" things in this part of his life. It is not surprising that cerebral palsied adolescents are often depressed, discouraged, resentful, and rebellious to a greater degree than many other young people during this stormy period of life (13).

Talk with the child's family; learn how they view his abilities as well as his disability. If he is not receiving speech correction, help locate this service. Give him praise for success and help in case of failure. Help him develop a sense of humor and a feeling of self-worth. Help him understand that he has responsibilities as well as privileges. In short, treat him as a person.

Aphasia

Aphasia refers to a language impairment caused by damage to the language area of the brain. Since cerebrovascular accident (stroke) is the most common cause of this disorder, and since stroke patients tend to be among the older population, we would not ordinarily expect to find an aphasic child in the regular classroom. Aphasia may result, however, from an external injury such as a blow on the head that caused brain damage. Such accidents can occur to a school-age individual; therefore, the possibility exists that this condition may be found in schools. The author knew a fourteen-year-old boy who was aphasic following a brain injury sustained in an automobile accident. After two years of hospitalization, physical, corrective, occupational, and speech therapy, he was enrolled in the regular junior high school. Without a sympathetic, understanding teacher and classmates, he would have been unable to function in this setting. He was fortunate. His teacher had unusual parental assistance and cooperation, and she had insight and understandings related to the problems of the handicapped that helped her assist him in many ways. Because, however, of the rarity of aphasia in the younger population, the problem is simply noted in this discussion.

The term *aphasia* refers only to the language impairment. There may or may not be motor involvement, depending on the extent of the cerebral insult. The patient's difficulty may lie primarily in his inability to encode language or it may be primarily in the decoding ability. He may be severely and permanently impaired both physically and linguistically or he may have only slight aphasic symptoms that may disappear within a few days, weeks, or months. Variations of severity lie between these two extremes.

Certainly brain damage may occur to the child prior to language learning, but these cases present an entirely different problem from the person who had acquired language prior to the cerebral insult. The neurologically impaired child was dealt with in the chapter on language disorders.

The Classroom Teacher and Children with Special Problems

If we resent having in our classroom a child with a special problem, if we feel insecure in attempting to work with the handicapped, if we are unable to overcome our feelings of undue sympathy, then perhaps we cannot be a good teacher for the handicapped. If, however, we can view each handicapped child as a person with a special disability and can seek ways to meet his special needs, then we will probably gain satisfaction from our experiences with the handicapped that we may never know in working only with the normal child—the one who may well succeed, even without our help.

Chapter 8

Hearing Problems

How does a classroom teacher respond to a child who habitually shows signs of inattentiveness, who is restless during story time, who is a "loner," or a "troublemaker," who consistently fails to follow instructions, or who makes unnecessary noise when he walks? If the teacher acts on instinct or applies stock judgments about such behavior, he may well conclude that the child is lazy, indifferent, or stupid, and his response to the child will convey this conclusion to him. Responses such as, "How could you make such a mistake?" or "Why don't you try?" or "Why won't you listen?" or "Are you too lazy to pick up your feet?" communicate to both the child and his peers that the teacher knows the source of the problem.

Many children in elementary schools suffer from some degree of hearing impairment, and this loss is often not recognized by the teacher or the parents. Estimates of the incidence of impaired hearing in the school population vary from 5 to 10 percent. Misunderstanding of their problem results in much needless difficulty with schoolwork. The problem of the hard-of-hearing child is one of social and educational significance. Specifically, it is the community that should feel a concern for the unfortunate financial and social effects of the retardation in school of children whose handicap has been neglected or not recognized. "Obviously, the repetition of grades is costly and in the long run, it is only a grossly superficial remedy which leaves the root of the problem quite untouched" (53).

The Nature of Sound

A simplified and perhaps rather superficial explanation of the nature of sound should help explain hearing. Sound is a vibration that has its origin in the vibration of a sound source, for example, strings of a violin or human vocal folds. The air itself is set in motion by the sound source as the at-rest position or air molecules are disturbed. As the disturbed molecules impinge upon each other, they create still further disturbance until a sort of chain reaction is set up. This process is perhaps analogous to a group of men standing in line when along comes a practical joker and shoves the one on the end (54). This knocks him into the man in front of him and so on down the line, with each man hitting the one in front of himself and then each one regaining his balance or original position. This pushing against each other in the case of men or molecules, causes a bunching up, and the regaining of their original position causes a thinning out. This compression and thinning out created sound waves. Each compression and thinning out constitutes one cycle, and the number of cyles that occur in one second denotes the frequency of the sound. Therefore, frequency is measured in cycles per second (cps). This is usually recorded in Hertz (Hz), which is the internationally standardized unit for measuring frequency.

The human ear is able to hear sound because its parts are set into motion by the vibrations of the air. Ordinarily we hear sounds conducted through the air. This process is known as air conduction. It is possible to hear via bone conduction, in which case the sound source transmits the vibrations directly to the bones of the skull and the air passageways are bypassed.

Frequency

Sounds differ from each other if their vibrations occur at different rates. This variance is frequency. Sounds of different frequencies are heard as different in pitch. A female voice is usually perceived as higher pitched than a male voice because of the differing frequencies of the different vibrating vocal folds. The sounds that the human ear can detect range from 20 to 20,000 Hz, but those that are important for speech occupy a much narrower band of about 250 to 3,000 Hz.

Intensity

Sound is energy. There is more energy in some sounds than in others. The term used to indicate the amount of energy in a sound is *intensity*, and the intensity of sound is perceived by the ear as *loudness*. The unit used to measure the intensity of sound is the decibel (dB). It is not an easy term to define, but basically it is a term used to describe the loudness or intensity of a sound, with zero dB representing the least sound pressure to which the best normal young adult ear can respond. A sound pressure over 85 dB is loud enough to damage hearing and those over 140 dB to cause the ear pain.

Most sounds, including those of speech, are complex sounds. They contain a large number of different vibrations occurring together, all of which vary in frequency. Generally speaking, vowel sounds are mainly composed of vibrations of low frequency, but some consonant sounds, especially the *s* and *f*, are composed primarily of relatively high-frequency vibrations.

The Hearing Mechanism

The ear is one of the most complicated organs in the body when studied in detail. For our purposes, it will be sufficient to understand it in terms of its three main divisions: the external ear, the middle ear, and the inner ear, which is well hidden in the temporal bone of the skull. See Figure 8.1.

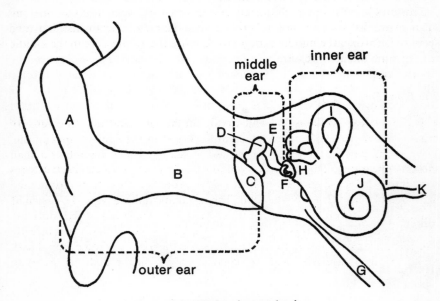

Figure 8.1. The hearing mechanism

A. pinna	D. malleus	H. oval window
B. external acoustic	E. incus	I. semicircular canals
meatus	F. stapes	J. cochlea
C. tympanic membrane	G. Eustachian tube	K. auditory nerve

The External Ear and the Middle Ear

The external ear is composed of the appendage on the side of the head that children learn to call "the ear" (A, pinna), together with the skin-lined canal (B, external acoustic meatus), at the inner end of which is the eardrum. The eardrum is really the middle ear, the drumhead of which is usually referred to as the drum (C, tympanic membrane). Inside the middle ear are three tiny bones called the ossicles, or the ossicular chain. One bone, the hammer (D, malleus) is attached to the drumhead and another, the stirrup (F, stapes), connects with the inner ear. The third or middle one, the anvil (E, incus), forms a bridge between the hammer and the stirrup.

Since these little bones are attached by means of ligaments and tiny muscles, they move when sound waves impinge upon the eardrum; thus they carry the vibrations across the middle ear to the inner ear, which contains the sensitive endings of the nerve of hearing. It is interesting to note that the little bones in the middle ear are fully grown at birth and are the smallest bones in the body. Diagrams of the middle ear may give an unrealistic impression of the size of the cavity—ten drops of water will completely fill it (12).

The middle ear is not a completely closed structure, since it has an opening through the Eustachian tube (G) to the nasopharynx. The Eustachian tube serves to ventilate the middle ear and to equalize the air pressure in the middle ear with the outside pressure.

The Inner Ear

The inner ear contains the end organ for hearing and also the sensory organ for balance (I), both of which are encased in the same bony capsule. The hearing part of the inner ear is the cochlea (J), which resembles a snail shell in appearance. This inner ear contains fluid matter in which are structures containing the nerve endings of hearing. In order for these to be stimulated there must be movement of the fluid. The mechanical force from the ossicular chain is applied to the fluid of the inner ear by the vibration of the footplate of the stapes, which moves in and out of the oval window that leads directly into the inner ear. Thus, these vibrations cause the hair cells to be stimulated, which in turn causes the hearing signal to travel via the auditory nerve to the brain.

Pathologies of Hearing

Hearing problems are described as (a) conductive, (b) sensorineural, or (c) mixed. A conductive type hearing loss is caused by some type of blockage or malfunction in the conductive mechanism (outer or middle ear); however, a sensorineural type loss is caused by actual damage to, or malfunction of, the end organ of hearing (within the inner ear) or the auditory nerve leading from the inner ear to the brain. In a mixed hearing loss, neither the conductive mechanism nor the sensorineural system functions normally.

An analogy could be drawn by visualizing a microphone placed in a container of putty. Although the microphone would not function properly, it would not be because the microphone was faulty, but because the sound waves could not get to it efficiently. This is the case with a conductive type hearing loss. If, however, there was no obstruction to the microphone and still the response was faulty, then the defect would be in the microphone itself. This is the condition in the case of a sensorineural loss. When there is both an obstruction to the microphone and a faulty microphone, we have a situation that is analogous to a mixed hearing loss.

Conductive Type Hearing Loss

Involvement of the external and/or middle ear results in a disruption of the conduction of sound waves. Something interferes with the conduction of the vibrations so that they do not reach the inner ear with their normal intensity. Hearing impairments resulting from this kind of loss are characterized by poor hearing in low tones and good hearing in high tones by air conduction, or a uniform loss of moderate proportions. The auditory nerve is functional, but the sound is not reaching it properly. This means that this type loss cannot make one deaf, since if the sound is loud enough, the bones of the skull will provide some vibration to conduct the sound to the hearing mechanism of the inner ear. This also means that such an individual is a good candidate for wearing a hearing aid, since all that he really needs is to have the sound reach his cochlea (which is functional).

This is the type hearing loss frequently encountered in schools. Much of it is transitory and associated with middle ear infections and malfunctions of the Eustachian tube. Much of it is remediable by medicine or surgery. More importantly, much of it is undetected. One of the common mistakes that laymen make is to assume that a person who speaks softly cannot have a hearing loss since "Hard of hearing people talk louder than normal hearing people." Speaking softly is often characteristic of one with a conductive type hearing loss. Sometimes a child, especially if he tends to be a shy, retiring child, will talk so softly that he can scarcely be heard in an ordinary classroom (12). He does so because he hears his own voice louder than he hears the speech of others. His own voice reaches his inner ear with normal intensity by bone conduction but, because of his faulty conductive mechanism he does not hear the speech of others as well. We tend to monitor our voices in terms of the loudness level of surrounding speech. The teacher will accomplish little by telling such a child to "talk louder" or to "speak up."

Involvements of the External Canal

Blockages can occur at the opening to the canal or in the canal itself. These can range from serious congenital closure (atresia), to the common problem of an excessive accumulation of ear wax (cerumen). The external ear is also subject to the same diseases that affect any other organ covered by skin such as impetigo, eczema, shingles, and fungus. Foreign bodies in the ear canal can also produce irritation of the tissues. Otologists have removed from ear canals almost any object light enough to be lifted above the shoulder and small enough to fit into the ear canal. Sometimes an object such as a bean, becoming warm and moist, will swell, causing pain as well as impaired hearing. The removal of such foreign objects should be accomplished by an otologist (13). Perhaps the most common cause of damage to the ear canal is the use of instruments such as hair pins or paper clips for purposes of removing wax or just scratching the skin of the canal. Infections of the external ear are called *external otitis.*

Involvements Affecting the Tympanic Membrane

The tympanic membrane may be damaged from without by sudden and extreme changes in the air pressure such as an explosion, or by puncturing by a sharp object introduced into the ear canal. Infections of the middle ear can cause the tympanic membrane to be forced either inward or outward. If infection in the middle ear results in sufficient fluid accumulation, the eardrum may be distended until it ruptures and the fluid escapes into the external canal. Blockage of the Eustachian tube may cause the air pressure in the middle ear cavity to be decreased so that the tympanic membrane is pushed inward by the outside air pressure.

Middle Ear Involvements

Many of the conditions of the eardrum are brought about by inflammation of the middle ear. This condition, called *otitis media,* is brought about by infection entering the middle ear via the Eustachian tube. Children have a high incidence of upper respiratory infections; likewise, they have more otitis media than do adults. The middle ear is connected to the air spaces in the mastoid area so that infections of the middle ear can spread to the lining of the mastoid cells. These cells then fill with fluid, and before the days of the "miracle drugs" the resultant mastoiditis was one of the dread diseases of childhood.

Otosclerosis is a fairly common disease among the Caucasian race, affecting the bony middle ear capsule. The cause is unknown, but an inherited predisposition seems to be present. In this disease the normal capsular bone is destroyed and replaced by a network of spongy weblike bone. Considering the tiny size of the middle ear, one can imagine the small amount of growth necessary to impede movement of the ossicles; yet it does not always produce a hearing loss. This is a disease of youth, occurring most frequently in adolescents and young adults. It occurs in about one of every eight white women and in about one of every fifteen white men. The incidence is about one in one-hundred in the black race, and little is known about its prevalence in the red, yellow, and brown races. The impairment of hearing is gradual and not complete. When the hearing loss first appears, the patient is often troubled by tinnitus (ringing in the ears). The loss is usually correctable by surgery.

Sensorineural Type Hearing Loss

A sensorineural type hearing loss is present when the vibrations of sound are properly transmitted through the ear canal, and from there across the middle ear to the oval window of the inner ear, but something "goes wrong" within the inner ear or along the pathway of the nerve to the brain. That is, the outer ear and middle ear are functioning normally, but there is some impairment of the inner ear or of the auditory nerve.

The child with this hearing loss is frequently misunderstood because of his inconsistent responses to sound. Although usually responding to his own name, this child may not understand when asked to do something, particularly if it is an unfamiliar task. His parents and teachers often accuse him of "not paying attention" and of "hearing only when he wants to." Actually, he may pay very close attention but hear only a jumble of sound that doesn't make sense. This jumble of sounds, quite understandably, makes more sense when the situation indicates what is to be done or indicates activities that are familiar. Since sensorineural type losses typically affect the higher frequencies, the child may hear predominantly low-pitched vowels in speech. Furthermore, since vowels carry little meaning, he obviously misses some of the meaning of speech.

In contrast to the child with middle ear impairment, the child with inner ear impairment has a much more serious speech problem. He may exhibit sound substitutions, distortions, and omissions in his speech. His voice may tend to be excessively loud, with a monotonous pitch pattern and a muffled voice quality. The chief methods to be used in correcting his speech are those which require the use of the visual, kinesthetic, and tactile senses as aids to such hearing as he may have (12).

Causes

The major causes of sensorineural hearing loss are advancing age, ototoxic drugs, and noise. By far the most common cause is advancing age. Indeed, the development of a certain amount of high-tone sensorineural hearing loss seems to be part of the natural course of growing older. Such hearing loss is known as presbycusis and obviously is not a problem of school-age children. Drugs, ranging from aspirin to dihydrostreptomycin, have been identified as ototoxic. The sensitivity of individuals to drugs and the amount and kind of drugs used determine the amount of damage done to hearing.

Noise-induced hearing loss is quite common. We are accustomed to background noise or masking that may block out the sound we wish to hear. This may do no more harm than to annoy us. Many of us, too, have experienced a noise so loud that we felt a temporary loss of hearing, perhaps accompanied by a ringing in our ears. This is known as "auditory fatigue," or temporary hearing loss. After a few hours, or by the following day, hearing is recovered. This temporary loss may be termed "fatigue," but somewhere injury begins, resulting in permanent noise-induced hearing loss. The injury may be a single, brief exposure to sound such as an explosion or a gun blast, and such an injury is called "acoustic trauma." The more common type of such loss is that caused by prolonged exposure to excessively loud noise, as that tolerated in some industries. This type hearing loss was formerly labeled "boilermaker's" deafness, but is now referred to as "noise-induced hearing loss." The loss begins around the frequency of 4,000 Hz and, without a hearing test, may go undetected until the damage has extended into the speech range.

Among children, sensorineural hearing loss is frequently associated with infectious diseases such as scarlet fever, meningitis, mumps, or some other disease of childhood that destroys hearing. Congenital deafness may be caused by almost any severe virus infection of the expectant mother, such as German measles during the early months of pregnancy. The Rh factor may also be associated with nerve type hearing loss. Heredity is a known factor in some cases, but unless both parents have true hereditary deafness, the chances that the children will become deaf are small (13).

Classifications

Basically there are two classifications for the hearing impaired: (1) *deaf* and (2) *hard-of-hearing*. The *deaf* are those for whom the sense of hearing is so impaired as to be non-functioning for the ordinary purposes of life. For children, this usually means that they were unable to learn speech through the avenue of hearing. The deaf may be subdivided into two groups. The *congenitally deaf* are those who were born without hearing. The *adventitiously deaf* are those who were born with hearing sufficient for the acquisition of speech but suffered severe hearing impairment later.

The *hard-of-hearing* are those for whom the sense of hearing, although defective, is functional with or without a hearing aid. This may be only a mild hearing loss or it may be so severe that the individual is severely auditorily handicapped. The classroom teacher would encounter few deaf children, but will expect to have some children with a degree of hearing impairment.

Clinical records indicate that many of the hard-of-hearing individuals of today may join the ranks of the deaf tomorrow. Fifty percent of adult deafness could have been prevented with proper medical attention in childhood. "The social and economic implications of these facts are sufficient to weigh heavily upon the conscience of all local and state authorities who have it in their power to improve the situation" (55).

Identification of Hearing Deficiency

Although children may exhibit symptoms of hearing loss, the only way that it can be determined for sure is through adequate testing. No whisper tests or watch-tick tests can do this, and schools should include identification audiometry as a part of the services to all children. This means that a program of hearing testing is carried on whereby the hearing of all children is screened routinely, and the hearing of all those failing the screening is tested further. Testing must be performed by a qualified person using a properly functioning audiometer. Identification without followup is worthless; therefore, remedial procedures must be provided for those needing such. Some diseases such as smallpox have been virtually wiped out through mass school vaccination programs; we have not made such giant strides with reference to hearing conservation programs.

The symptoms of hearing deficiency are so varied that no one symptom would be interpreted as indicating the possibility of a loss, but if a child exhibited a number of such symptoms he should be tested, whether he is in the grade to be screened that year or not. Some of these symptoms are:

1. Lack of attention to casual conversation.
2. Frequent requests to repeat what has been said.
3. Frequent earaches and complaints of ear difficulties.
4. Tendency to be withdrawn and lack of desire to be involved in social activities.
5. Difficulty in articulating certain speech sounds.
6. Frequent confusion as to what has been said.
7. Constant visual scanning of the speaker's face.
8. Verbal directions ignored consistently.
9. Consistently turning the head to one side when paying attention to the teacher or another student.
10. Close observation of the face of the teacher.
11. Reading disability.
12. Spelling errors.
13. Frequent colds with ear discharge.

14. Spells of dizziness or head noises.
15. Daydreaming.
16. Difficulty in taking dictation.
17. Indifference to music.

BUT, the most important thing to remember about symptoms is that WAITING FOR THESE SIGNS IS WAITING UNTIL MUCH TOO LATE!

The Role of the Classroom Teacher

It is generally recognized that the child with a hearing loss, which is about one of every twenty children, is at a disadvantage in learning situations; it is less commonly realized that he is at a disadvantage socially and emotionally. Consider the following situations. The chatter of other children goes unnoticed, and the child may become depressed and lonely. At the same time he may become sensitive and suspicious, wondering if the other children could be talking about him. The teacher may call on him in class, and he does not answer because he does not hear. Another child nudges him; he looks toward the teacher, who now repeats the question. This time the child answers; he is able to "hear" what is said because he is looking at the teacher's face. The teacher assumes that he is not paying attention and reprimands him for his poor attitude.

Even though a teacher may know of a child's difficulty, he may find it irritating to have to repeat things to him or he may feel that it is a burden to have to give special help. When one realizes that the child affects all persons in his environment in much the same way, it becomes evident that he needs special help with the problems of building self-confidence and of socialization. These children have a special handicap, since they wear no crutches, braces, or bandages; they do not advertise their defect. Bewilderment and frustation may become their reactions.

It is often assumed that the hard-of-hearing child has a lower native intelligence than the normal hearing child because of his educational retardation. The more he fails or drops behind the more he, his teachers, and his parents become convinced that he is dull; but research does not support this assumption. Studies indicate that the hard-of-hearing child is comparable to the normal child in native intelligence, that he is retarded in language development and scores lower on verbal intelligence tests than the normal child, and that he is below the normal child in academic achievement. "The fact that he is comparable to the normal hearing child in intelligence, yet definitely below him in achievement, points to an unsolved educational problem" (56).

Studies reveal that the hard-of-hearing child is slightly more introverted, slightly more submissive, and develops an inferiority complex more often than the normal hearing child. Because of this apparent stupidity, his indifference to his environment, his inattentiveness, his introversion and feelings of helplessness, the hard-of-hearing child is often misunderstood and consequently mistreated. Since attitudes toward other persons and toward society as a whole are formed largely during childhood, serious damage can result from such misunderstandings. Each time the teacher fails to recognize the hard-of-hearing child's handicap and blames laziness or lack of intelligence for lack of success, he is instilling a spirit of resentment in the child.

The teacher, however, cannot be expected to understand or help the acoustically handicapped child unless the impaired condition is known. Furthermore, he cannot assume the existence of that condition simply because the child presents personality problems. The imperative need for identification becomes obvious.

The classroom teacher can do much to help the hearing-handicapped child to live with others successfully. Through the classroom experiences and general climate, he can help the child attain a sense of social competence in the normal school environment. Although the hard-of-hearing child is likely to withdraw from others, the teacher can draw him into group living by giving him duties and helping him to accept responsibilities shared by the hearing members of the class.

A healthy attitude toward himself and his handicap is not enough, however. The teacher can aid the child in developing language abilities by encouraging him to converse with others and by motivating him to use speech and to take part in the classroom activities. He can make sure that the child's experiences are fairly broad in nature. In addition, the teacher can encourage him to take part in playground activities and to read widely.

If there is a speech correctionist in the school, he or she and the classroom teacher have a dual role to fill in teaching the hard of hearing. First, together they may be able to help the child make an adequate social adjustment with his classmates. Second, they may be able to help the child improve his speech. Third, they may be able to provide the needed academic supplement to the regular school program.

If the child wears a hearing aid, the correctionist may be able to help the teacher provide opportunity for him to display it to the class. Perhaps this can be integrated with a unit on communication comparing the aid to a telephone; or perhaps it can be worked into a unit on health, learning to take care of the ears.

It may be possible to help the other children experience how it feels to have defective hearing by having the children cover their ears and try to understand whispered directions; or perhaps the teacher can play children's records at the lowest possible volume and have them guess what's playing. A game can be made of having the children listen to a clock tick and see how far they can move away from it and still hear it tick. Seeing that they don't all cease to hear at the same spot will help them to realize that hearing in normal ears varies.

Speech reading can be correlated with phonics. Games such as "What sound do you see now?" will help children learn to correlate visual clues with auditory ones. Even the morning roll call may be done in this way without voice. The English language presents many difficulties to the deaf and hard-of-hearing because it is not phonetic. There are also many words that are homophonous; that is, they look alike on the lips as: *mama* and *papa*. Cognate sounds such as *s* and *z*, *f* and *v*, *p* and *b* are differentiated only through the use of hearing, rather than through the use of sight.

The classroom teacher may be able to assist the speech clinician by listing new words or expressions introduced into the classroom conversation. In this way, the new words and expressions may be corrected as to pronunciation, given in auditory training and speech reading, as well as explained with respect to correct usage in language development.

The teacher and the speech correctionist can help the parents of the hearing-handicapped child by passing along various types of information to them. Often the parents of deaf children do not know that the child can be trained in language and speech. It should be remembered, however, that the child's first and most important teachers are his parents, and one of their most significant functions is the guidance of his emotional development. The teacher has no control over the type of treatment that the child had in his preschool years. Some parents who have good mental health themselves and constructive attitudes toward their child's hearing loss will have been able to do much in preparing the young hard-of-hearing child for school.

The teacher and the correctionist can learn much from the parents about the kind of preschool experiences that the child has had. They can determine if his parents understood the importance of (a) having him within easy seeing-hearing distance when talking to him and not shouting to him when he was in another room; (b) talking to him a great deal; (c) speaking clearly and distinctly when talking to him; (d) using the language that they would use if they were speaking to any other two-year-old; (e) explaining his handicap to friends, relatives, and playmates and not being secretive about it. If his parents have done these things, then fortunate is the child and also his teacher.

If, however, the child did not have parents with such insights, the teacher is faced with the problem of providing the child with many of the experiences that will compensate for his early lack of learning experiences.

Although the classroom teacher will not be expected to be a "special teacher," he should understand that most speech correctionists have had training in teaching speech reading and otherwise working with the hard-of-hearing, and thus are able to provide the classroom teacher with assistance in the form of suggested procedures to help the hearing handicapped child.

Suggestions to Teachers of Hearing-Handicapped Children

1. Provide the hearing-handicapped child with preferential seating. Assign his seat near where you will be most of the time, away from open windows and doors, with his back to the light, and with his better ear (if one is better) toward you. This means providing him with the most advantageous place to take advantage of both speech reading and his residual hearing.
2. Be sure he can see your lips and face.
   a. Don't talk while writing on the chalkboard.
   b. Don't stand with your back to the window while talking. Shadows and glare make it difficult to see your lips (speech read).
   c. Don't seat him so that he faces the light.
   d. Keep your hands and books down from your face while speaking, and do not move your head. Don't use gestures alone to indicate thought, etc. Use gestures naturally.
   e. Stand fairly still while speaking with light on your face.
   f. Be sure you have his attention before giving assignments.
   g. Don't exaggerate or "mouth" words. Exaggerated mouth movement makes speech reading difficult. Speak naturally and avoid using loud speech.
3. Encourage him to watch the speaker's face.
   a. Encourage him to watch your lips when you are talking to the class.
   b. Permit him to turn around and face the class so that he can see the lips of the reciter.
   c. Permit him to move his seat whenever class activity is in different parts of the room. If he is given such a privilege with respect and obligation, he will not abuse the privilege, and other children will not resent it.
4. Be sure that he is understanding what is being said and done.
   a. Help the child understand the meanings of similar words by using them in sentences. Many words look alike on the lips and can be distinguished only by context.
   b. Do not proceed too far in your discussion without asking or making sure that he understands. If he does not understand, restate the

material in a different way. Perhaps he was not familiar with the key words.

c. Remember to watch the child for signs of lack of comprehension. Recall that when repetition does not help you should rephrase the material.

d. Emphasize what is being taught by writing on the chalkboard, but remember not to talk while writing. Names of people and places are difficult for the hard-of-hearing person to understand. It is well to place new vocabulary words on the board and to discuss the new material from this vocabulary.

e. Assign another child to help the hard-of-hearing child get the correct assignments.

5. Help the child work out his own measuring stick for monitoring the loudness of his own voice. The teacher can take a few minutes now and then to help him recognize the loudness level that he should maintain.

6. Have the child read ahead of the material discussed in class. This helps him to understand the vocabulary.

7. Stress clear enunciation on the part of yourself and the other pupils. Remember to speak a little louder than you may for the average child, but not unnaturally loud.

8. Remember that the hard-of-hearing child requires special help in all language activities, such as reading and spelling. His hearing handicap directly affects his language background; therefore, encourage him to take an active interest in reading, spelling, social studies, and other language arts.

9. Teach the child to use the dictionary with skill and to learn the pronunciation system so that he can attack and pronounce new words.

10. Stimulate his residual hearing and add rhythm to his speech by encouraging him to participate in musical activities such as vocal music and choral reading.

11. Encourage participation in extracurricular activities. Help him to feel a part of the group. Hard-of-hearing individuals tend to withdraw from the group.

12. The hearing-handicapped child becomes more easily fatigued because of the close attention he must give. He needs sympathetic understanding. Alternate activities that require close attention with those in which he can relax.

13. Try to prevent colds, throat and nose complications, running ears, etc., in the child with a hearing impairment. If they do occur, see that he receives medical attention.

14. Give parents an accurate account of the child's educational achievement. They should know the truth.

15. Try to keep the hard-of-hearing child on the academic level with his classmates.
16. Find a time to explain the problem of the hard-of-hearing child to the other pupils. Point out that special considerations to be shown him should be given without calling attention to his impairment.
17. Allow him to recite and to read orally just as you do any other member of the class.
18. If he is attending speech-reading lessons, allow some other children to attend a lesson with him. This fosters their understanding.
19. Furnish the speech correctionist with academic-content words to be used in speech-reading lessons. This aids the child and his teacher in the academic program.
20. Be sure that his hearing is checked at least once each year.
21. Above all, help him to understand and to acknowledge his hearing problem. This is one of the most important aspects of any handicapped child's problem, but it is especially important for the hard-of-hearing child. If he learns early in life to say when meeting a stranger, "I am hard-of-hearing and so may not understand what you say," he will meet people on common ground with no apologies and nothing to hide. How much better than pretending to hear, appearing dull, and having strangers dislike and misunderstand the odd behavior!

Fortunate, indeed, is the hard-of-hearing child who finds himself in the classroom of a sympathetic, understanding, and insightful teacher who is willing and capable of making adjustments within her classroom to help ease the school situation for him.

The hard-of-hearing child in her class is truly an integral part of the group. He knows he has certain privileges which the others do not have but he does not abuse them because he has learned to respect the teacher and classmates in the manner in which he is respected. . . . By setting up a permissive atmosphere in her classroom for the hard-of-hearing child, the group absorbs her philosophy and in turn consciously or unconsciously passes on its knowledge and understanding to others. (57)

References

1. V. Anderson and H. Newby. *Improving the Child's Speech*. New York: Oxford University Press, 1973.
2. W. H. Perkins. *Speech Pathology*. Saint Louis: C. V. Mosby Co., 1971.
3. C. Van Riper. *Speech Correction, Principles and Methods*. Englewood Cliffs N.J.: Prentice-Hall, Inc., 1972.
4. P. Moore and D. Kester. Historical notes on speech correction in pre-association era. *Quarterly Journal of Speech*, Dec., 1938, 24:642–54.
5. R. Mackie and L. Dunn. *State Certification Requirements for Teachers of Exceptional Children*, Office of Education Bulletin, No. 1. Washington: U.S. Government Printing Office, 1954.
6. W. Johnson. *Children with Speech and Hearing Impairment*. Office of Education Bulletin, No. 5. Washington: U.S. Government Printing Office, 1959.
7. American Speech and Hearing Association. *1974 Directory*. Danville, Ill.: Interstate Printers and Publishers, 1974.
8. G. Garrison *et al.* Speech improvement. *Journal of Speech and Hearing Disorders*, Monograph Supplement No. 8, July 1961, pp. 78–92.
9. P. Phillips. Factors related to teacher's opinions and understandings concerning speech handicapped school children. Unpublished doctoral dissertation. Auburn University, Alabama, 1966.
10. M. Himman. The teacher and the specialist. *National Education Association Journal*, Nov., 1960, 59:24–25.
11. Committee on the Mid-Century White House Conference. Speech disorders and speech correction. *Journal of Speech and Hearing Disorders*, June, 1952, 17:129–37.
12. J. Eisenson and M. Ogilvie. *Speech Correction in the Schools*. New York: The Macmillan Company, 1971.
13. W. Johnson *et al. Speech Handicapped School Children*. New York: Harper & Row, 1967.
14. J. Sheehan and M. Martyn. Spontaneous recovery from stuttering. *Journal of Speech and Hearing Research*, Mar., 1966, 9:121–35.
15. H. Davis and R. Silverman. *Hearing and Deafness*. New York: Holt, Rinehart, & Winston, 1970.
16. S. Duker. Goals of teaching listening skills in the elementary school. *Elementary English*, Mar., 1961, 38:170–74.
17. M. Bonner. A critical analysis of the relationship of reading ability to listening ability. Unpublished doctoral dissertation. Auburn University. Alabama, 1960.

18. M. Moss. The effect of speech defects on second grade reading achievement. *Quarterly Journal of Speech*, Dec., 1938, 24:642–54.

19. T. Eames. The relationship of reading and speech difficulties. *Journal of Educational Psychology*, 41, 1950.

20. M. Jones. The effect of speech training on silent reading achievement. *Journal of Speech and Hearing Disorders*, Sept., 1951, 16:258–63.

21. R. Ham. Relationship between misspelling and misarticulation. *Journal of Speech and Hearing Disorders*, Aug., 1958, 33:294–97.

22. P. Phillips. *Classroom Speech Problems*. Auburn, Ala.: University Printers, 1973.

23. M. Quintillian. *Institutes of Oratory*. London: G. Bell & Sons, 1892.

24. D. McNeill in F. Smith and G. Miller, editors. *The Genesis of Language*. Cambridge, Mass.: M.I.T. Press, 1966.

25. M. Lewis. *How Children Learn to Speak*. New York: Basic Books, 1959.

26. H. Myklebust. *Auditory Disorders in Children*. New York: Grune & Stratton, Inc., 1954.

27. L. Mayer. *Notebook for Voice and Diction*, Dubuque, Iowa: W. C. Brown, 1960.

28. G. Fairbanks. A theory of the speech mechanisms as a servosystem, *Journal of Speech and Hearing Disorders*, June, 1954, 19:133–39.

29. H. Winitz. *Articulation Acquisition and Behavior*. New York: Appleton-Century-Crofts, 1969.

30. K. Snow. Articulation proficiency in relation to certain dental abnormalities. *Journal of Speech and Hearing Disorders*, Aug., 1961, 24:209–12.

31. J. Yedinak. A study of the linguistic function of children with articulation and reading disabilities. *Journal of Genetic Psychology*, Mar., 1949, 74:23–59.

32. R. Everhart. The relationship between articulation and other developmental factors in children. *Journal of Speech and Hearing Disorders*, Dec., 1953, 18:332–38.

33. R. FitzSimons. Developmental, psychosocial, and educational factors in children. *Child Development*, Dec., 1958, 29:481–89.

34. C. Weaver *et al*. Articulatory competence and reading readiness. *Journal of Speech and Hearing Research*, June, 1960, 3:174–80.

35. R. Sommers *et al*. Effects of speech therapy and speech improvement upon articulation and reading. *Journal of Speech and Hearing Disorders*, Aug., 1961, 26:27–38.

36. E. Zedler. Effect of phonic training on speech sound discrimination and spelling performance. *Journal of Speech and Hearing Disorders*, June, 1956, 21:245–50.

37. O. W. Nelson. An investigation of certain factors relating to the nature of children with functional defects of articulation. *Journal of Educational Research*, Nov., 1953, 47:211–16.

38. G. Siegel. Experienced and inexperienced articulation examiners. *Journal of Speech and Hearing Disorders*, Feb., 1962, 27:28–34.

39. N. Wood. *Delayed Speech and Language Development*. Englewood Cliffs, N.J.: Prentice-Hall, Inc., 1964.

40. M. Berry and J. Eisenson. *Speech Disorders.* New York: Appleton-Century-Crofts, Inc., 1956.
41. E. A. Davis. *The Development of Linguistic Skill in Twins, Singletons with Siblings, and Only Children from Age 5–10.* Minneapolis: University of Minnesota Press, 1937. In Berry and Eisenson (38).
42. T. Bangs. Evaluating children with language delay. *Journal of Speech and Hearing Disorders,* Feb., 1961, 26:6–18.
43. S. Beasley. *Slow to Talk.* New York: Bureau of Publications, Teachers College, Columbia University, 1956.
44. T. Battin and O. Haug. *Speech and Language Delay: A Home Training Program.* Springfield. Ill.: Charles C. Thomas Publishing Company, 1970.
45. R. West. An agnostic's speculation about stuttering, in J. Eisenson, *Stuttering: A Symposium.* New York: Harper & Row, 1958.
46. J. Eisenson. A perseverative theory of stuttering, in J. Eisenson, *Stuttering: A Symposium.* New York: Harper & Row, 1958.
47. R. Webster. Decrease in stuttering frequency as a function of continuous and contingent forms of auditory masking. *Journal of Speech and Hearing Research,* Mar., 1970, 13:82–86.
48. P. Glauber. The psychoanalysis of stuttering, in J. Eisenson, *Stuttering: A Symposium.* New York: Harper & Row, 1958.
49. I. H. Coriat. The psychoanalytic conception of stuttering. *The Nervous Child,* 2, 1943.
50. W. Johnson. *An Open Letter to the Mother of a Stuttering Child.* Dannville, Ill.: Interstate Printers and Publishers, 1962.
51. E. J. Brutten and D. Shoemaker. The modification of stuttering. Englewood Cliffs, N.J.: Prentice-Hall, Inc., 1967.
52. D. Fox. *Clinical Management of Voice Disorders.* Lincoln, Neb.: Cliffs Notes, Inc., 1974.
53. H. Davis and R. Silverman. *Hearing and Deafness,* New York: Rinehart & Winston, 1964.
54. H. Newby. *Audiology.* New York: Appleton-Century-Crofts, 1972.
55. L. Dicarlo. Program for children with impaired hearing. *Elementary School Journal,* Nov., 1948, 49:160–67.
56. L. Dahl. *Public School Audiometry.* Danville, Ill.: The Interstate Publishers and Printers, 1949.
57. E. Eagles *et al. Hearing Sensitivity and Related Factors in Children.* Pittsburgh: University of Pittsburgh Graduate School in Public Health, 1963.

Glossary

Adventitious: Acquired, not present at birth.

Air conduction: The transmitting of sound waves to the cochlea by way of the outer and middle ears.

Aphonia: Loss of speech; voicelessness.

Assimilation: The modification of a speech sound by the influence of a sound or sounds uttered in close sequence with it.

Audiometer: An instrument for measuring objectively the acuity of hearing.

Auditory memory span: The ability to recall immediately sound sequences. May be tested clinically by having subject repeat sequence of vowel sounds or repeat digits.

Bone conduction: The transmitting of sound waves or vibrations to the cochlea via the bones of the skull.

Central Nervous System: C.N.S.; the brain and the spinal cord.

Cleft Lip: Chiloschisis; hare lip; a congenital cleft of the upper lip; may extend into the roof of the mouth; may be on one side (unilateral) or on both sides (bilateral).

Cleft Palate: Uranoschisis; a congenital cleft of the roof of the mouth; may involve only the soft palate; may involve both soft and hard palate; may extend through the gum ridge; may be unilateral or bilateral.

Congenital: Existing at birth; may be hereditary or the result of pathology following conception of the embryo. (Always refers to disease, deformity, or deficiency.)

Consonant: A speech sound, voiced or voiceless, in which the chief characteristic is a non-musical friction noise generated by driving the expired air through so narrow an opening as to raise its pressure and thus its speed, creating sound waves.

Cyst: A sac with a distinct wall, containing fluid or other material.

Differential Diagnosis: A discriminating diagnosis aimed at distinguishing a given case of disorder from one or more other disorders.

Diphthong: A vowel-like sound made while the articulators are in rapid movement from the position for one vowel to that of another.

Eustachian: The tubular passageway connecting the pharynx with the middle ear.

Evaluation: An assessment of a given case in order to determine the diagnosis of the problem, the prognosis for remediation, and therapeutic management indicated.

Fibroma: A benign tumor composed principally of fibrous connective tissue.

Fricative: Speech sounds made by forcing the airstream through a narrow opening, for example, making audible high-frequency sounds, *th*, *v*, *h*, *s*.

Functional: Not organic; referring to behaviors or reactions that are not caused by physical structures or conditions; learned.

Guttural: Pertaining to the throat; throaty.

Hematoma: A cyst, or swelling, caused by bleeding under conditions that prevent its escape from the site of the hemorrhage.

Idioglossia: Any unique speech code developed spontaneously by a child and not resembling the language of his family; usually intelligible only to one or two siblings or close associate. (Not to be confused with a code learned in order to achieve secrecy such as "Pig Latin.")

Kinesthetic: Muscle sense.

Larynx: The voice box.

Laterality: Sidedness, as handedness, eyedness, footedness.

Lisping: Defective utterance of sibilant sounds, *s*, *z*, *sh*, *zh*; usually refers to defective *s* and *z*.

Malocclusion: Failure of the teeth of the lower jaw to meet those of the upper jaw properly.

Nasal: Pertaining to the nose.

Nasal Cavity: The passageway from the outer air to the pharynx via the nostrils.

Nodule: A small node; a small aggregation of cells.

Organic: Not functional; caused by physical structures or conditions.

Palate: The roof of the mouth, including the anterior portion (the hard palate) and the posterior portion (the soft palate, or velum).

Palsy: Paralysis.

Papilloma: A wartlike tumor.

Pathology: The study of disease; the state of being diseased or a condition caused by disease; the explanation of some disturbance of function in terms of the absence or defect of the parts responsible for the function.

Pharynx: The throat; the part of the respiratory tract that extends from the nasal cavity to the larynx.

Phonate: To produce voice by means of laryngeal vibrations.

Phoneme: The smallest differences in a language that serve to differentiate meanings within the language, for example, *b*, *d*, *k*.

Plosive: Speech sounds made by impounding the airstream momentarily until considerable pressure has been developed and then suddenly releasing it, as in *p* or *d*.

Polyp: A pedunculated nodule.

Posterior: Back; pertaining to the back part or position of the body or of an organ.

Psychogenic: Originating in, produced by, or caused by a mental reaction, as opposed to physiogenic.

Rehabilitation: Restoring of a function or skill that has been lost, or the development of one that is absent but normally should be present.

Resonance: The modification of the laryngeal tone by passage through the chamber of the throat and head so as to alter its quality.

Sibilant: High-frequency fricatives, *s*, *z*, *sh*, and *zh*.

Tactile: Sense of touch.

Therapy: Any treatment, medication, training, exercises, or other management of a case designed and intended to bring some abnormal condition closer to normal.

Tongue Tie: Abnormal shortness of the frenum of the tongue.

Trachea: The windpipe; the respiratory passageway from the larynx to the bronchi.

Trauma: Produced by violent mechanical causes such as falling, crushing, stabbing, etc.; somewhat figuratively, serious mental shock.

Vowel: A voiced speech sound resonated and emitted through the mouth with the structures positioned so that no friction noise is created by the airstream.

Bibliography

ANDERSON, V., and NEWBY, H. *Improving the Child's Speech.* New York: Oxford University Press, 1973. This book was written especially for the classroom teacher. It emphasizes the importance of the classroom teacher in the speech education of all children and of those with speech disorders in particular. Materials are simply presented but with enough explanation to make them useful.

BANGS, T. *Language and Learning Disorders of the Pre-Academic Child: With Curriculum Guide.* New York: Appleton-Century-Crofts, 1968. The fairly extensive curriculum guide at the conclusion of this book is perhaps the most useful part of it to classroom teachers. It is especially appropriate for teachers in early childhood education.

EGLAND, G. *Speech and Language Problems.* Englewood Cliffs, N.J.: Prentice-Hall, 1970. Written especially for classroom teachers, this book deals with speech problems in a limited way. The most extensive treatment is of the problem of stuttering. It also deals with such problems as the quiet child and the one who talks excessively. It also contains a number of case descriptions that could be helpful in visualizing some of the problems discussed.

EISENSON, J., and OGILVIE, M. *Speech Correction in the Schools.* New York: Macmillan, 1971. This book contains an excellent presentation of the impact that speech problems in the schools have on the child's entire educational experience. It also describes the various speech problems to be encountered in the schools.

EVANS, B. *Visible Phonics and Articulation.* Mobile, Ala.: University of South Alabama Bookstore, 1973. This is a small book presenting a phonic approach to teaching sounds and is written especially for use by classroom teachers. It contains the English speech sounds, a description of how each is made, spelling rules, word lists, pronunciation rules, and articulation drills.

JOHNSON, W. (ed.). *Speech Handicapped School Children.* New York: Harper & Row, 1967. This is a rather long and detailed presentation of various speech problems, with special emphasis on the responsibility of schools for providing remedial speech services. It would be a good source book for teachers interested in learning more about a specific speech problem.

MCNEIL, D. *Acquisition of Language: The Study of Developmental Psycholinguistics.* New York: Harper & Row, 1972. For the student who wants a concise, yet authoritative and fairly thorough, study of how language is acquired, this book would serve as an excellent text.

NEWBY, H. *Audiology*. New York: Appleton-Century-Crofts, 1972. This is an excellent source for information concerning the hearing mechanism, how hearing can be tested, the various problems to be found, and the need for hearing testing. It is factual, informative, and authoritative, yet fairly simply presented.

VAN RIPER, C. *Teaching Your Child to Talk*. New York: Harper & Row, 1950. This book was written especially for lay reading and gives a very readable and easily understood explanation of how children learn to talk. There are numerous suggestions to parents relative to facilitating speech.

————. *Speech in the Elementary Classroom*. New York: Harper & Brothers, 1955. This small book contains a concise presentation of the need for training in oral communication. Emphasis is placed on speech improvement, with the inclusion of sample speech-improvement lessons.

————. *Speech Correction, Principles and Methods*. Englewood Cliffs, N.J.: Prentice-Hall, 1972. This book gives a fairly detailed description of the various speech problems and their therapeutic management. It is intended for the speech pathologist, but is understandably written and may serve as a source book for classroom teachers who want to learn more about specific problems and their therapeutic management.